FERTILITY AND NUTRITION

DR. KAMINI RAO
ROHIT SHELATKAR

STARDOM BOOKS

www.StardomBooks.com

STARDOM BOOKS, LLC
112, Bordeaux Ct,
Coppell, TX 75019

FIRST EDITION MARCH 2025

STARDOM BOOKS

A Division of Stardom Alliance
112, Bordeaux Ct,
Coppell, TX 75019
www.stardombooks.com

Stardom Books, United States Stardom Books, India

FERTILITY AND NUTRITION/
Dr. Kamini Rao, Rohit Shelatkar

p. 187
cm. 13.97 X 21.59

Category: Health & Fitness/ Fertility / Nutrition

ISBN: 978-1-957456-37-9

Table Of Contents

Prelude

Anyone from the older generation will tell you much has changed in the past fifty years. In today's fast-paced world, our lifestyles have undergone drastic changes, which, in turn, are majorly affecting our health.

Rapid urbanization and the IT revolution have undoubtedly translated to more car commutes, desk jobs, and longer work hours –forcing millions into a more stressful yet sedentary lifestyle with erratic eating and sleeping habits. There has been an explosion in the incidence of chronic lifestyle diseases such as obesity, diabetes, cardiac issues, cancer, and fertility issues.

Over 95% of the world's population has health problems, with over a third having more than five ailments.

-The Lancet

In the context of fertility issues, it is safe to say that poor dietary habits, lifestyle diseases, environmental toxins, genetic changes, sexually transmitted infections, unfettered use of emergency contraception, and deferring parenthood are among the major causes of infertility. Even worse, these issues are compounded by intensive work conditions, stress, exposure to pollutants and toxins, alcohol and drug abuse, and the rising incidence of obesity.

Today, as many as one in seven couples trying to have a baby will experience infertility.

-National Institutes of Health

The most common contributing yet modifiable factor to this trend is our diet. Over the last few decades, our eating habits have changed drastically, with our diets becoming almost unrecognizable compared to those of our grandparents and great-grandparents. We witness a transition from freshly prepared traditional, staple foods to processed foods with high content of sugar, salt, trans fat, and little or no nutrients.

We have come a long way in the last 50 years in terms of what we eat, how we exercise, how we do business, and how we treat ailments. It begs the question, what will our lives be like in the next 50 years? It is time we put a saddle on our lifestyle and dietary habits.

Instead of popping umpteen pills for umpteen different problems, it's time we track back to nature and turn to the dynamic duo – food and exercise. Fresh foods loaded with nutritional elements are bound to keep us healthy; exercise keeps us fit and even helps manage stress. These should be your go-to remedies!

Thomas Edison famously said, "The doctor of the future will give no medicine but will instruct his patient in the care of the human frame, in diet, and the cause and prevention of disease."

A surefire way of promoting better health and curbing diseases starts at the base, which means ensuring better health for upcoming generations. So then, do we look at the hen or the egg? ***Fertility and Nutrition Book is both.*** A healthy mother means a healthy offspring. This book gives you an overview of the right kind of diet and lifestyle, to help you prepare for pregnancy, enhance fertility, and maintain a healthy weight and nutritional status during pregnancy. This not only creates a supportive and healthy home for your infant's nine month stay, but it also determines the long-term health of your bundle of joy.

1. Pregnancy should be a planned event, not an accident.

2. Pre Pregnancy Checkup

3. A visit to the doctor should be done before falling pregnant.

4. Nutritional Corrections should be before pregnancy

5. Pregnancy is not an illness. It's a natural phenomenon of reproduction. For mothers who are happy and enjoy pregnancy, the baby grows better.

Foreword

By Dr Rustom Phiroze Soonawala.
MD., F.I.C.O.G, F.R.C.S., F.R.C.O.G. **Obstetrics and Gynaecologist, Padma Shri Awardee**

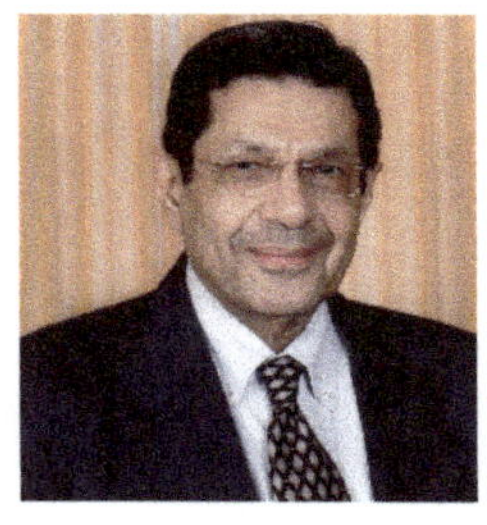

Can my diet affect my chances of becoming pregnant? - this is a universal concern among both women grappling with infertility and healthy women hoping to become pregnant. **Do I have to eat for two?** - the most widespread misconception that pregnant women have. **How do I lose weight after having a baby?** - a post-pregnancy cliche. Not only are these common concerns that women face at various stages of their lives, but they are also questions that are put to almost every gynecologist daily.

Infertility in a couple can stem from several problems. Modern medicine offers state-of-the-art assisted conception technology; however, this is not the only solution to infertility. Sometimes, the solution lies in a modest diet and lifestyle optimization. Regarding pregnancy, we often underestimate the power that lies in the hands of nutrition. The impact of nutrition on the life-long health of the child and mother is often overlooked. Breastfeeding ensures the proper nourishment of newborns; however, breastfeeding mothers often forget to nourish and nurture their bodies.

Infertility & Nutrition is a scientific compilation that brings these aspects to light and addresses allies' issues, concerns, and queries. Throughout the book, Dr. Kamini Rao and Rohit

Shelatkar provides specific practical advice that will inspire readers to take charge of their diets and lifestyles. It also helps gynecologists to advise their patients on these aspects.

In today's fast-paced world, several diseases occur due to poor lifestyle and diet choices. With their quick fixes and fad diets, Charlatans of the healthcare industry seem ever intent on beguiling the public. This book is the need of the hour to help both the common stay on the right track.

To my family, friends, colleagues, and all the couples struggling and striving in the hope of having children.

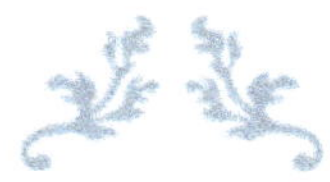

Anna was a career-oriented, ambitious lady in her early thirties. Like most working couples, she and her husband decided to settle down in their respective careers before having children. Now that they were comfortable with their jobs, the couple made a joyful decision of having children. Months and years of disappointment finally pushed them to visit a gynaecologist and find out if there was an issue with either of them.

It was after a few doctor visits, the couple came to understand that many aspects of their life – the years of stress they had taken on at work, the reckless, sedentary lifestyle they led, the poor food choices they made and the age at which they decided to have children – all of these determined whether or not they could have children. As a matter of fact, even their body weight wasn't to their advantage. Anna was puzzled, it had never hit her that so much can affect her fertility. Can it really? Read on to find out….

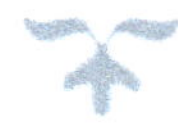

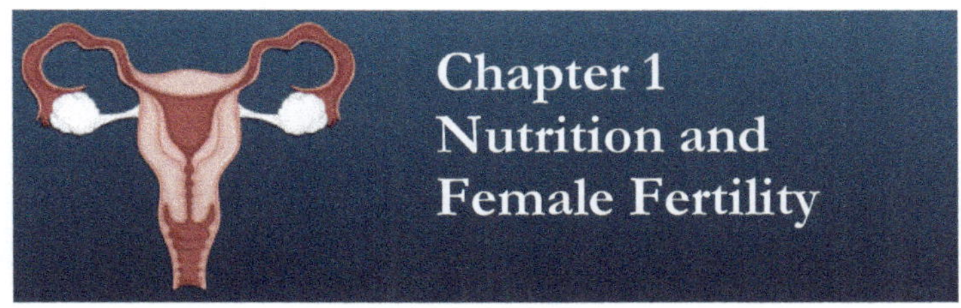

Chapter 1 Nutrition and Female Fertility

Parenting begins before conception: Yes! Emerging research reveals that parental influences begin even before conception.[1] Science continues to reveal more and more evidence that maternal age, diet, and nutritional status, among others, significantly impact several fertility aspects and the quality of eggs, which can impact future offspring.

Ageing: Only Wine Gets Better

Ageing is related to a drop in the ovarian reserve of eggs and a decrease in the quality of eggs that is up for grabs.[2] It is essential to understand that the quality of an egg is a vital element in the ability to conceive. The quality of the egg lies chiefly on its genetic material - deoxyribonucleic acid, popularly known as DNA.[3] DNA, along with some proteins, tightly packed like a spool of yarn, form chromosomes. Each chromosome has bodyguards called telomeres (protective caps of chromosomes). Ageing shortens the telomeres, affecting an individual's chromosomes and, therefore, the fertility potential.[4]

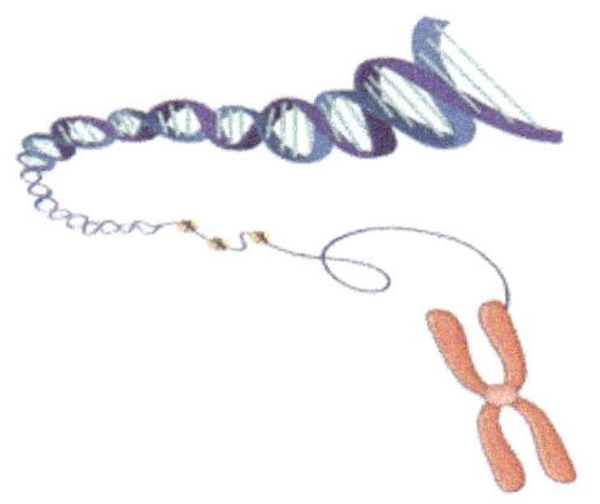

Not just ageing, telomere shortening can be influenced by physical activity, body mass index, smoking, chronic inflammation, oxidative stress, dietary antioxidants, and vitamin deficiencies.[4]

Stress: It's Just a Mess!

Most of us deal with the immense stress of the 21st-century lifestyle. Unfortunately, it belongs to the list of factors that contribute to infertility. Psychological stress can negatively impact the maturation of the oocyte (egg). De-stressing can aid in increasing conception rates.[2]

Weighing It Out: Impact of Body Composition on Conception

Underweight and, to a greater degree, overweight and/or obesity are related to an enhanced risk of infertility.[5]

While mitochondria are found in every cell of the body, each egg has over fifteen thousand mitochondria, which is ten times more than any other cell in our body.[3]

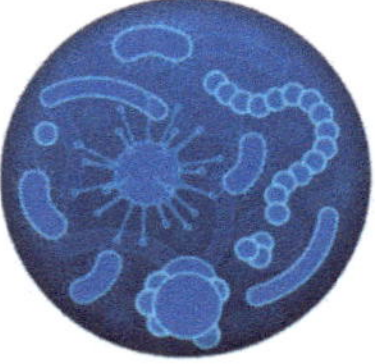

An egg requires massive energy to process chromosomes correctly and execute all other processes necessary for proper maturation. All these are supported by the powerhouses called mitochondria. The mitochondrion, stated, is a miniature powerhouse that converts nutrients into a form of energy that the cells of the body can use.[3] Embryogenesis (the development of a fertilized egg) is also an energy-demanding process, and oocyte-derived mitochondria are required to support it.[1]

A meager food intake, strong dietary restrictions, and a general lack of nutrients not only cause a loss of both body weight and physical performance but also delay puberty and lengthen the postpartum interval to conception. Moreover, they are also known to lower reproduction-related hormone (gonadotropin) secretion, and this alters ovulation cycles (the process by which eggs are released from the ovary for fertilization) and is thereby linked to increased infertility.[6]

Very slim women (BMI, body mass index <20 kg/m^2) have a 38% higher risk of infertility than women with average body weight (BMI 20–24 kg/m^2). This is simply because reproduction involves much more energy expenditure for females than males. As a protective mechanism against undernutrition, women's reproductive capacity is closely linked to their nutritional status. No wonder eating disorders that lead to loss of weight are related to either reduced or hampered ovulation. Even with a small percentage of weight gain, one can easily hope for the return of ovulation.[5]

Besides energy balance, poor intake of proteins, minerals, and vitamins is associated with reduced reproductive performance.[6] Overweight and obesity can harm normal endocrine function, paving the way for fertility disorders. Overweight and obesity not only interfere with ovulation, but they also affect implantation (attachment of the fertilized egg to the uterine lining). This means an increased risk of miscarriages and more disappointments with *in-vitro* fertilization (IVF) procedures.[5]

Let's understand this better: the expanded adipose tissue seen in obese individuals leads to a disturbance in the production of substances called adipokines (an increase in leptin and resistin production and a decrease in adiponectin production). The crosstalk among these adipokines, the brain (hypothalamus, pituitary), ovaries, oocytes, embryo, and the female reproductive tract directly and indirectly affects female reproduction.[7]

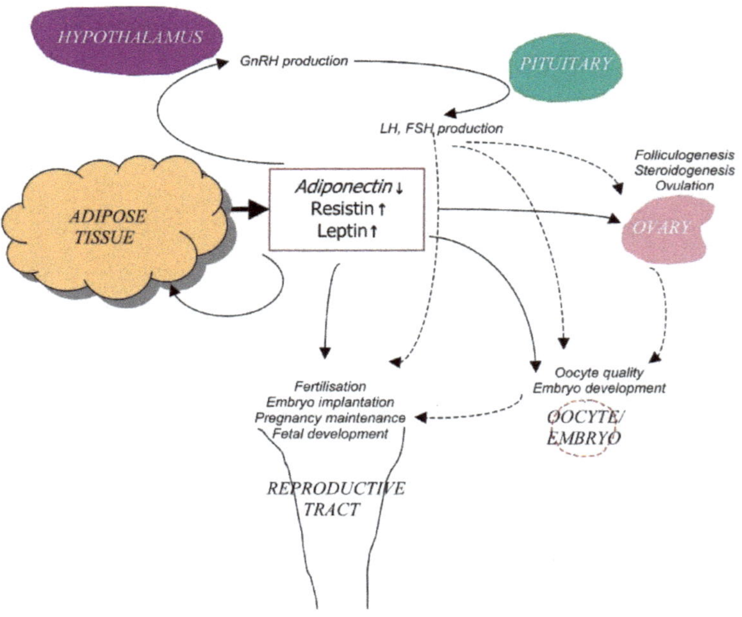

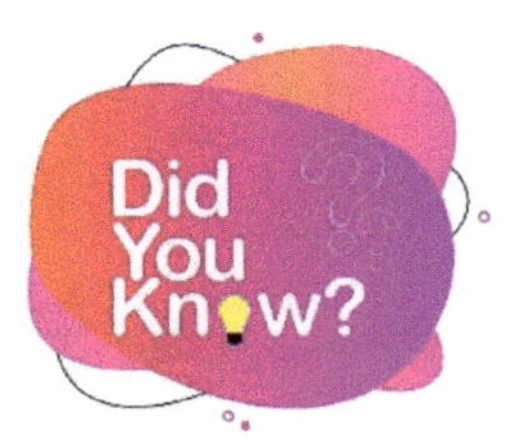

B.....P.....A? More like **Be 'P**'har **A**way. You heard it right: if you plan to conceive, you better avoid bisphenol A (BPA). This toxin meddles with the body's hormones and has thus earned the reputation of an endocrine disruptor. Research has proven that BPA promotes obesity and compromises egg quality and fertility in females. Unfortunately, even after conception, BPA is detrimental, as it may lead to miscarriages by making the uterine lining less receptive.

7
OTHER

We are exposed to BPA more commonly than we think. Bisphenol A leaches from reusable bottles and plastic containers (polycarbonate plastic #7), especially for hot food or liquids. We all enjoy piping hot coffee from reusable, plastic travel mugs and often use plastic blenders to blend hot soups. Next time, think twice. Not just that, beware if your water bottles have been sitting in hot places for a long time — such as in a car sizzling in the sun! Bottled and canned sodas, soft drinks, and alcohol are also significantly associated with increased BPA levels in the body![8,9]

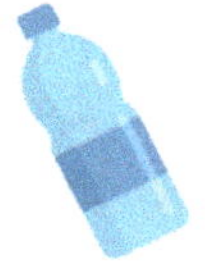

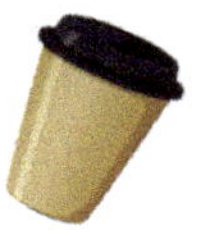

Carbonless paper receipts from gas stations, grocery stores, and restaurants contain BPA, which is absorbed through the skin.[8]

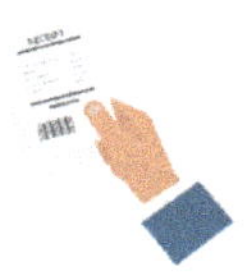

Heads up! BPA-free is not a good idea either. Manufacturers replace BPA with closely related compounds. Be it BPA or its chemical cousins – bisphenol S and bisphenol F – the harm is the same.[3]

How to Steer Clear of BPA?

The good news is much can be done to reduce and avoid exposure to BPA. The place to begin is your kitchen: swap plastic items (especially those that come in contact with heat) with glass or stainless steel. Minimise the use of canned and bottles food and drinks. If there is an absolute need for plastics, opt for polypropylene or High-density polyethylene (HDPE) plastic. Also, practice hand-washing after handling paper receipts.[3]

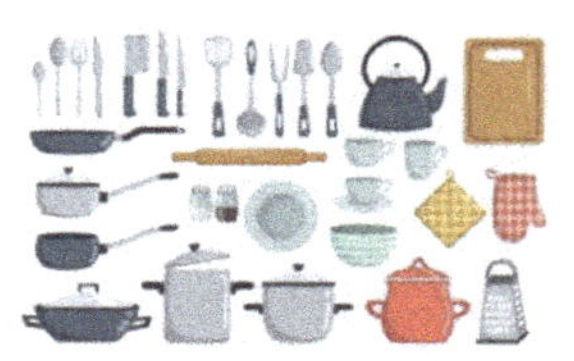

Kitchenware to be aware.

- Reusable food storage containers
- Microwave-safe utensils
- Reusable bottles and cups
- Colanders
- Blenders

Pssssttt…….

It's not just BPA that is an endocrine disruptor, phthalates, used in plastics, cleaning products, nail polish, and perfumes, also belong to this class of chemical criminals. A phthalate known as Di-2-ethylhexyl phthalate (DEHP) is also found in processed food![3]

Role of Foods and Nutrients in Preconception Health

Maternal nutrition affects oocyte provisioning; the maternal environment influences oocyte stores of mitochondria and metabolites.[1]

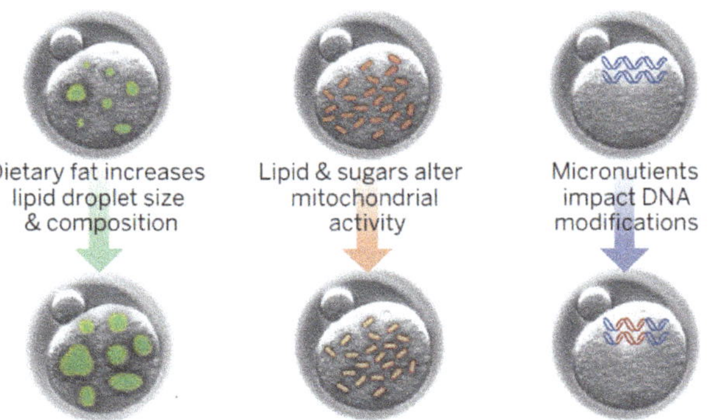

It had been hypothesized that several ovulatory disorders are due to the effects of carbohydrate intake on glucose metabolism. In line with this, science has unearthed that total carbohydrate intake and the glycaemic load of the diet are linked with infertility caused by ovulation disorders.[5] A higher dietary glycaemic load (GL) is linked to elevated fasting glucose levels, hyperinsulinemia, and insulin resistance, elevating free insulin-like growth factor (IGF-I) and androgens. Consequently, endocrine disturbance and oocyte maturation defects are witnessed.[2] Likewise, in women who have not given birth earlier, a similar relationship has been spotted between the glycaemic index (GI) of food and infertility.[5] In healthy women, it has been shown that the consumption of animal protein is linked with an increased risk of infertility and the consumption of vegetable protein with a lower risk of infertility.[2] In this regard, a 5% energy swap from animal protein to energy from vegetarian protein leads to a staggering 50% reduction in the risk of infertility due to ovulation disorders.[10]

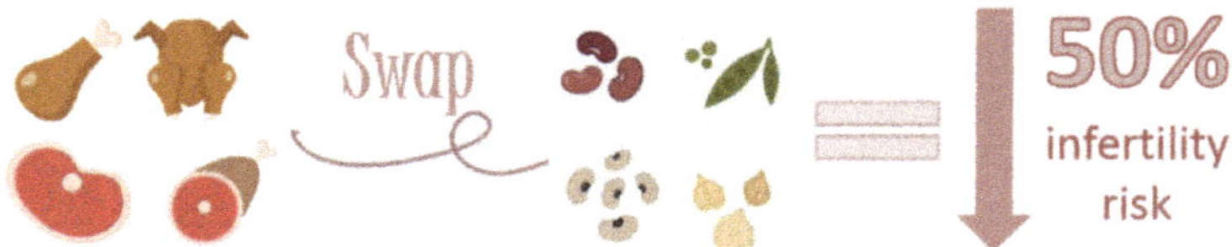

This phenomenon can be attributed to the beneficial effects of vegetable protein on insulin resistance. Moreover, vegetarian protein also keeps a check on IGF-I levels.[5] In women treated for infertility, higher dairy protein intake (≥5.24% of total energy intake per day) has been seen to cause lower antral follicle counts, reflecting poor fertility potential.[10]

High-fat intake increases testosterone levels in healthy women by a minimal degree and also adversely affects embryo quality.[10] Higher intake of polyunsaturated fatty acids (PUFAs), specifically an omega-3 fatty acid called docosapentaenoic acid, has demonstrated a lower risk of anovulation (absence of ovulation resulting in infertility).[2,10] In women with polycystic ovary syndrome, trans-fatty acids heighten the risk of ovulatory infertility.[10]

Higher testosterone levels in women=Risk of infertility

Preliminary research indicates that choosing fat-laden milk over skimmed milk is beneficial, as the palm transonic acid present in milk aids in the reduction of insulin resistance. However, we await further research in this niche domain.[5]

Oxidative stress is an imbalance between free radicals and antioxidants in the body; it can lead to cell and tissue damage. It can cause variations at the DNA level and thereby impact reproductive capacity.[2]

↓ Beneficial antioxidants
↑ Harmful free radicals
Oxidative stress

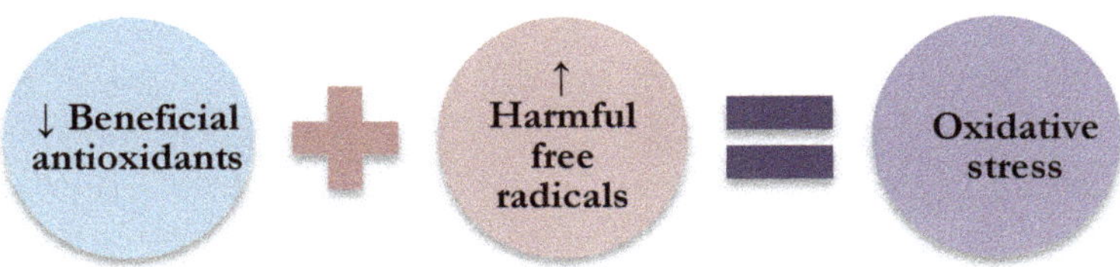

Daily consumption of more than a serving of citrus fruits rich in beta-cryptoxanthin (an antioxidant) decreases the risk of endometriosis (abnormal growth of endometrium lining that can cause infertility) by a fourth. Among women undergoing IVF, a higher intake of whole grains providing nutrients supporting antioxidant defense such as phytic acid (a unique natural substance found in plant seeds), vitamin E, and selenium during the pre-treatment period has demonstrated a higher probability of live birth.[10]

Genetically modified food can potentially risk fertility, as it influences endocrine metabolism.10

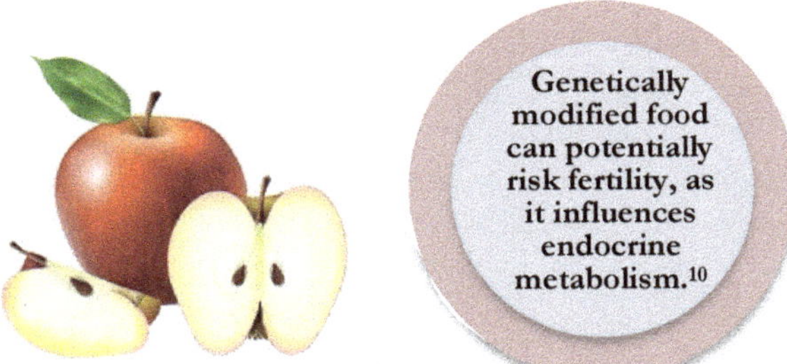

High intake of non-haeme iron, viz. iron of plant origin (such as whole grains, legume seeds, and certain vegetables), can also help reduce the likelihood of infertility due to ovulatory disorders.[5] Folic acid enhances embryo quality, improves pregnancy chances, and reduces ovulatory infertility risk.[2] Similarly, high levels of vitamin B12 are also linked to better embryo quality.[1]

Non-nutritive substances

Tobacco smoking damages the quality of eggs, markedly affects the reproductive health of women, and adversely impacts IVF outcomes. Smoking is also linked with a rapid decline in ovarian reserves, delayed conception, and a heightened risk of spontaneous miscarriage, as well as a lower success rate from assisted reproductive technology (ART). Heavy alcohol consumption (four or more drinks per week) indirectly affects fertility through nutritional or secondary health disorders and may also adversely affect IVF outcomes. Last but not least, high caffeine consumption (≥500 mg caffeine) delays conception, and even a 100 mg caffeine intake can increase the risk of pregnancy loss.[2,11,12]

Key Takeaways

- Age, stress, diet, and nutritional status have a major impact on several fertility aspects and the quality of eggs, which can impact future offspring.
- Underweight and, to a greater degree, overweight and/or obesity are related to an enhanced risk of infertility.
- Chemicals such as bisphenol A and phthalates present in plastics adversely impact fertility.
- Several foods and specific nutrients play a role in female fertility.

Nutrition and Fertility Word Sleuth

Here's a word search to delight the detective in you. Hunt for ten words that you came across while reading this chapter.

```
G V Q L T A V U I F S A D G R E E
J Q R K J E D L W S I C G J B C X
T L M X P T L J L R R S R E I N Q
N I L U S N I O D N T X U E S A R
T G P W R A Z N M N F C K H P T H
Q H Z W A X O I A E P M G N E S N
P B G X O H V D R H R H U P N I W
H L T I C U I X T O M E G A O S C
Y B S O E X D H X M H O V H L E H
Q G T Q O W A Y Y S Q E K P A R T
L I L I Y L R Y B E P G Q B D S A
M P T Q A I O E P K X Q O E T S G
P N S T A R F F D J K D Q D R E Z
A P E O G R I U Z N S T F A C R O
U J A O R W Y L Z U U Z G D A T S
G L Y C A E M I C I N D E X Z S N
H A N G Q O Z M R X L A K T U M N
```

Answers

ANTIOXIDANTS OMEGA TELOMERE

BISPENOL A PHTHALATE INSULIN RESISTANCE

UNDERWEIGHT STRESS

MITOCHONDRIA GLYCAEMIC INDEX

References

1. Lane M, Robker RL, Robertson SA. Parenting from before conception. *Science.* 2014:756–760.
2. Silvestris E, *et al.* Nutrition and female fertility: An interdependent correlation. *Front. Endocrinol.* 2019;10:346–358.
3. Rebecca Fett. It Starts with the Egg: How the Science of Egg Quality Can Help You Get Pregnant Naturally, Prevent Miscarriage, and Improve Your Odds of IVF. 2nd edn. Franklin Fox Publishing: New York, 2014.
4. Vasilopoulos E, Fragkiadaki P, Kalliora C, *et al.* The association of female and male infertility with telomere length (Review). *Int J Mol Med.* 2019;44(2):375–389.
5. Szostak-Węgierek D. Nutrition and fertility. *Med Wieku Rozwoj.* 2011;15(4):431–436.
6. The ESHRE Capri Workshop Group, Nutrition, and reproduction in women. *Human Reproduction Update.* 2006;12(3):193–207.
7. Mitchell M, Armstrong D, Robker R, *et al.* Adipokines: Implications for female fertility and obesity. *Reproduction.* 2005;130(5):583–597.
8. University health news. Available at: https://universityhealthnews.com/daily/nutrition/5-alarming-sources-of-bpa-exposure/. It was accessed on 29 July 2019.
9. Today health. Available at: https://www.today.com/health/bottled-water-hot-plastic-may-leach-chemicals-some-experts-say-t132687. Accessed on: 29 July 2019.
10. Çekici H. Current nutritional factors are affecting fertility and infertility. *Ann Clin Lab Res.* 2018;6(1):225.
11. Firns S, Cruzat VF, Keane KN, *et al.* The effect of cigarette smoking, alcohol consumption and fruit and vegetable consumption on IVF outcomes: a review and presentation of original data. *Reprod Biol Endocrinol.* 2015;13:134.

12. Oostingh EC, Hall J, Koster MPH, *et al.* The impact of maternal lifestyle factors on preconception outcomes: A systematic review of observational studies. *Reproduc Biomed Online.* 2019;38:77–94.

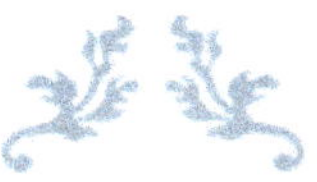

Let food be thy medicine and medicine be thy food.

–*Hippocrates*

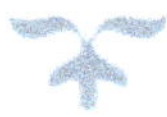

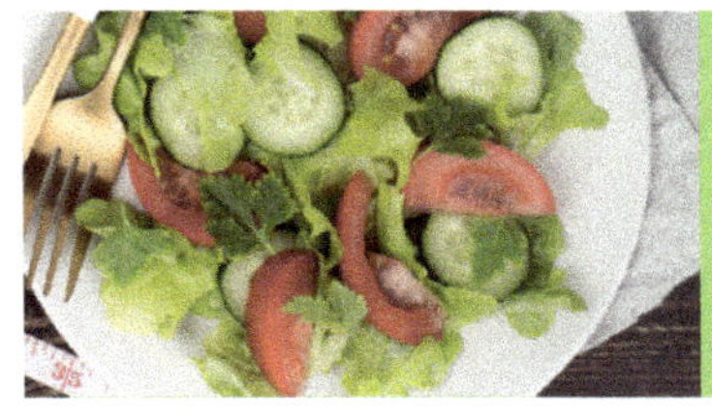

Chapter 2 Female Fertility: Diet, Lifestyle, and Exercise

Undoubtedly, you might be confused about what to eat, what not to eat, whether there's a perfect diet to boost fertility, or how to lose weight.... Worry not; you are on the right page!

Balanced Diet

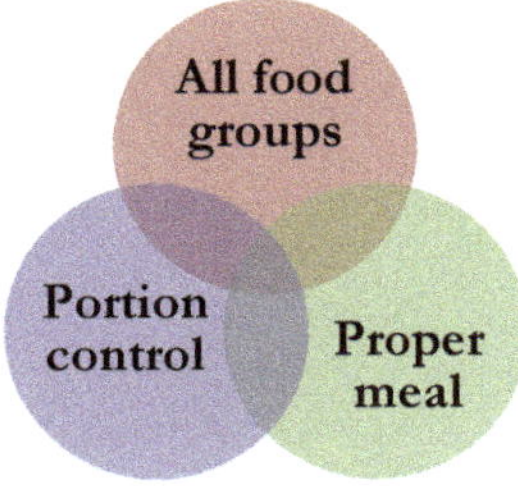

A well-balanced diet is the backbone of a healthy lifestyle. A balanced diet ensures the consumption of all food groups in the right proportions; this ensures optimal intake of all nutrients.[1] The 'Healthy Eating Plate' can be used as a guide for eating healthy, balanced meals.[2]

Healthy Eating Plate[2]

Use healthy oils (like olive oil & canola oil) for cooking, on salad, and at the table. Limit butter & avoid trans fat.
Eat plenty of fruits of all colours. Whole fruit is better than juice.
The more veggies and more variety you eat, the better. Non-starchy veggies are better, so French fries don't count!
Drink water, tea or coffee with little or no sugar. Limit milk/dairy to 1-2 servings/day and avoid sugar-laden beverages.
Choose whole grains (whole-wheat bread, whole-grain pasta, brown rice). Limit refined grains (while bread, white rice).
Opt fish, poultry, beans and nut; limit red meat nad cheese. Avoid bacon & processed meat.

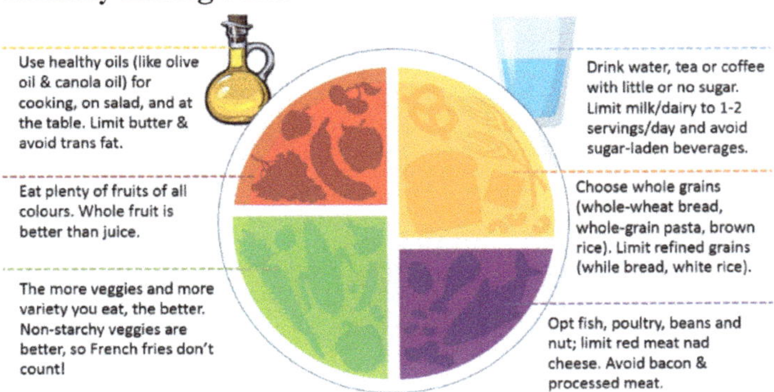

Regarding fertility, certain specific healthy balanced diets have been in the spotlight, and rightly so.

Mediterranean Diet

The Mediterranean diet, or MedDiet, is inspired by the nutritional regimens of people of Greece, Southern Italy, and Spain.[3]

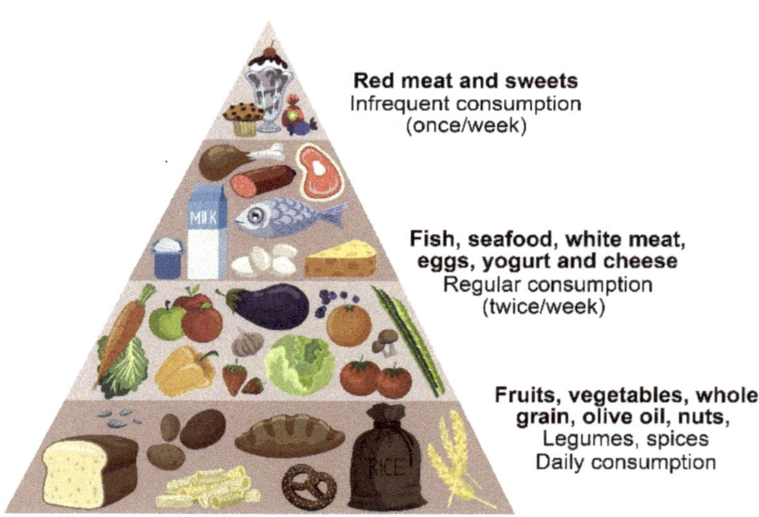

It's easy to understand why the MedDiet is on the list for those trying to conceive. Science says it's positively related to folate and vitamin B_6 levels in the blood and with follicular fluid levels and a 40% increase in the possibility of pregnancy after intracytoplasmic sperm injection (ICSI)/IVF treatment.[3,4]

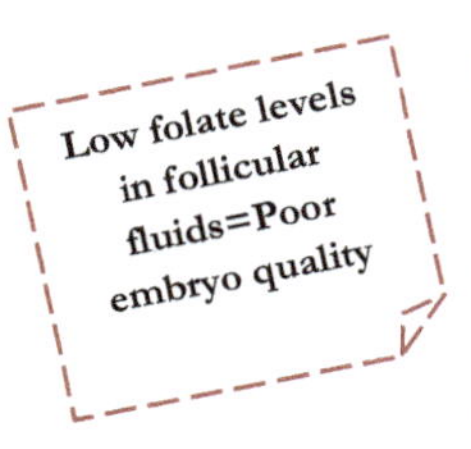

Fertility Diet

Designed to boost fertility, the fertility diet is similar in many ways to the MedDiet. Whipping up food as per this diet means:[5,6]

Selecting slow carbs and not no carbs: Carbohydrates rich in fibre: Whole grains, vegetables, whole fruits, and beans have a high glycaemic index.

Guess What?

Remember the bodyguards of chromosomes, the ones that reduce with ageing? Yes, telomeres! The MedDiet also helps protect them! Here are some other tips to preserve telomeres:[7–9]

Choose:

- ✓ Whole grains, legumes, nuts, and seaweed
- ✓ Healthy fats (from avocados, fish, and nuts)
- ✓ Flax seeds, chia seeds, sesame seeds
- ✓ Kiwi, black raspberries, lingonberry, red grapes
- ✓ Broccoli, sprouts, tomatoes, olive fruit
- ✓ Fibre-rich diet

Stay away from:

- ✗ High calorie intake
- ✗ Sugar-laden foods and beverages (e.g. soda, soft drinks, fruit-flavoured drinks, sports drinks, energy drinks, and diet soda)

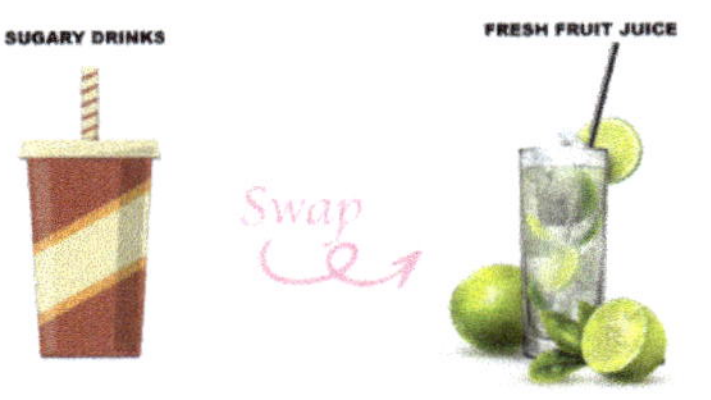

Choosing veggie protein: Swap a serving of meat daily with beans, peas, soybeans, tofu, or nuts.

Steering clear of trans fat: Trans fats are artery-clogging fats known to harm the heart and blood vessels. But here is something we don't know: they also threaten fertility.

Using more unsaturated vegetable oils: Monounsaturated and polyunsaturated fats favor fertility by enhancing insulin sensitivity and reducing inflammation. Cut back on saturated fat and consume vegetable oils, nuts, seeds, and fish such as salmon and sardines.

Opting for whole milk: Whole milk aids in the reduction of insulin resistance, a property that skimmed/lean milk lacks.

Packing plenty of iron from plants: Additional iron from plant sources, including whole-grain cereals, spinach, beans, pumpkin, tomatoes, and beets, is beneficial. Vitamin C-rich accompaniments such as citrus-based drinks, bell-peppers, and berries enhance iron absorption.

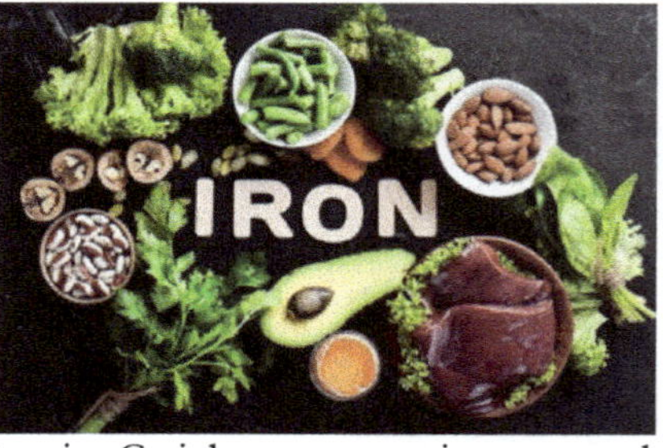

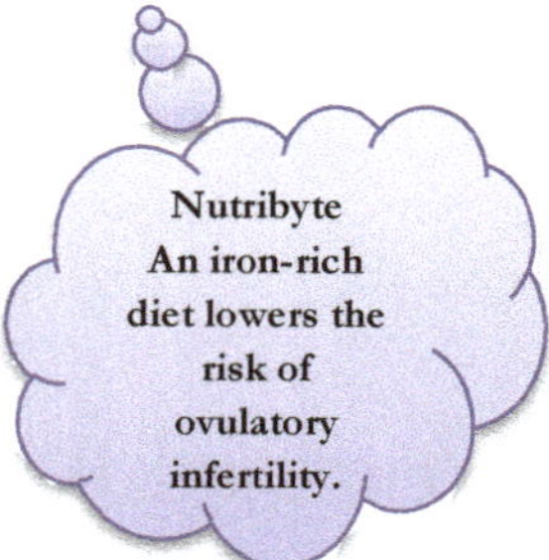

Remember, folic acid supplementation (400 mcg/day) is a must and should be during preconception (read more in the chapter on neural tube defects).

Bottoms up? Only with water: Water is the best beverage for hydration. The harms of alcoholic and caffeinated beverages have already been covered previously. But bear in mind that sugar-laden drinks and sodas are no better: they are carb-criminals that appear to promote ovulatory infertility.

Last but not least, **hustle the muscle**. An ideal body mass index (BMI) enhances fertility.

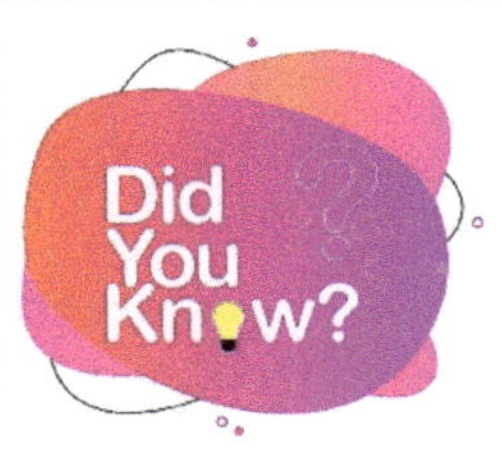

Exercise and yoga can also boost fertility.

Being in the healthy weight range reduces the risk of infertility and improves the chances of conceiving spontaneously, as well as with assisted reproductive technology (ART).[10]

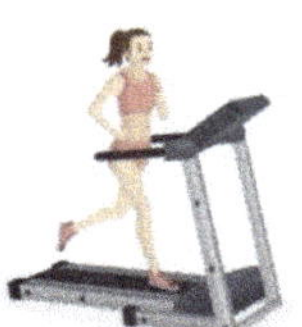

As per international guidelines, at least 30 minutes of moderate-intensity physical activity, such as brisk walking, gardening, or dancing, is recommended on most or preferably all days of the week. Vigorous activity, such as running, fast cycling, or fast swimming, should be performed weekly if feasible.[10]

Don't be a brat. Burn that fat!

Overweight or obese adults benefit from better health and fertility through modest weight loss. They must stick to 225 to 300 minutes of moderate-intensity weekly exercise (about 35 to 45 minutes daily).[10]

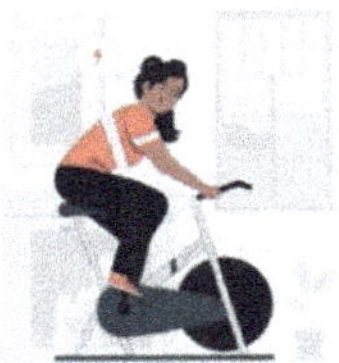

Be cautious. Too much very high-intensity exercise may reduce fertility and the chances of conceiving with ART. So, avoiding very high-intensity exercise while trying for a baby is a good idea.[10]

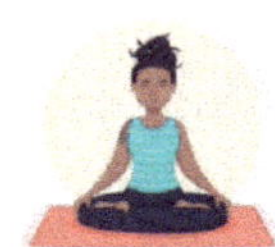

Exercise the Body and the Mind

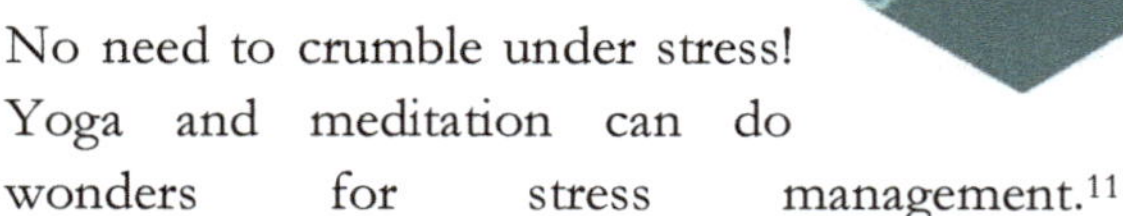

No need to crumble under stress! Yoga and meditation can do wonders for stress management.[11]

Why all the noise about the fertility diet, anyway? In 2007, Harvard researchers demonstrated that women with ovulatory infertility had a staggering 66% drop in the risk of ovulatory infertility and a 27% lower likelihood of infertility from other causes by following this diet compared to women who didn't follow the diet.[6]

The recommendations that ensue the fertility diet are aimed at preventing and reversing ovulatory infertility. While the diet itself doesn't guarantee a pregnancy any more than assisted reproduction, it has several advantages – it is accessible and available to everyone, has no side effects, sets the stage for a healthy pregnancy, and forms the foundation of a beneficial eating strategy for motherhood and beyond.[5]

In a nutshell, a woman's fertility is improved by consuming a well-balanced diet based primarily on foods of vegetable origin, legume seeds, whole-grain cereal products, and a choice of vegetable fats, delivering large amounts of monounsaturated fatty acids.[4]

Micronutrients: Mini Magicians

Micronutrients include vitamins and minerals; they are required in minute quantities but play crucial roles at various stages of fertility. Let's have a look.[12]

Micronutrient	Role in female fertility
Folate	Oocyte quality, maturation, fertilisation, implantation
Zinc	Ovulation, menstrual cycle
Vitamin A	Oocyte quality, development of fertilized egg (blastogenesis)
Zinc and certain B-vitamins	DNA synthesis (fundamental to the development of oocytes)
Folate and zinc	Apoptosis (viz. normal cell death; essential for regulation of follicle atresia, degeneration of corpus luteum, and endometrial shedding)
Folate; vitamins B_6, B_{12}, and D; iron	Homocysteine metabolism (adequate level linked to better success in infertility treatments), inflammation, oxidative stress, embryogenesis
Vitamins C, E, and A	Fight against reactive oxygen species (ROS caused by stress, smoking, alcohol use, extremes of body weight, exposure to environmental toxins, and advanced maternal age) that impair oocyte maturation, ovulation, luteolysis, and follicle atresia.

There is limited scientific evidence on the influence of micronutrient status on female fertility; there is a lack of human studies on the subject. Nevertheless, it is worth noting that women who struggle to conceive do have lower-than–recommended levels of certain micronutrients.[12] Here are the critical issues unearthed by studies so far:

- Insufficient vitamin B_{12} levels are seen in more than half of infertile women.[13]
- Infertile women seem to have lower vitamin B_6 levels than fertile women.[14]
- Conception is less to occur if there is inadequate vitamin D intake or if there is deficiency or inadequacy of serum 25-hydroxyvitamin D.[15]
- Vitamin D deficiency is also linked to conditions that impair fertility (such as polycystic ovarian syndrome) and can adversely affect the outcomes of infertility treatments.[16,17]
- Total serum antioxidant status is lower in women with PCOS and in the peritoneal fluid of women with idiopathic infertility.[18]
- Inadequate selenium level increases the risk of luteal phase deficiency, in which insufficient progesterone secretion by the corpus luteum makes the endometrium less receptive to implantation.[19]
- Serum and follicular fluid selenium, zinc, and copper levels are significantly lower in women undergoing IVF compared with controls (healthy, non-pregnant women of the same age).[12]
- Women undergoing IVF show increased oxidative stress (known to enhance iron absorption), reflected by higher follicular fluid levels of aluminum and iron compared to controls.[12]

- Women receiving IVF also have lower antioxidant levels (vitamins A and C and glutathione peroxidase) and show more damage due to oxidants (lipid peroxidation in serum and follicular fluid) compared to controls.[12]

Since adequate micronutrient levels are essential for fertility (oocyte quality, maturation, fertilisation, and implantation) and deficiencies are noted in women with infertility, it appears rational to presume that restoring micronutrients to recommended levels may positively impact fertility.[12]

While healthy diets improve fertility, consumption of such diets may sometimes be challenging, even with easier access to fresh, nutritious foods. The preconception diet can be adversely affected by social, economic, educational, ethnic, cultural, and genetic factors, leaving many women of childbearing potential with a suboptimal micronutrient status.[12]

In such instances, micronutrient supplementation before conception may help restore micronutrients to recommended levels and, thereby, potentially positively impacting fertility.[12]

Micronutrient Supplementation to Enhance Fertility

Multiple micronutrients (MMN) supplementation with 800 μg of folic acid for at least one month before conception and throughout the first trimester has been shown to significantly increase the number of confirmed pregnancies and cut down the time to conception when compared with supplementation with trace elements (copper, manganese, zinc, vitamin C). Folic acid supplementation has also been reported to increase fecundability (i.e., the probability of conceiving during a single menstrual cycle with unprotected intercourse).[12]

Vitamin D supplementation in women with PCOS and hypovitaminosis D may improve menstrual frequency and metabolic disturbances. In comparison to no supplementation, vitamin E supplementation has been shown to significantly increase endometrial thickness in women with unexplained infertility undergoing controlled ovarian stimulation.[12]

Supplementation with MMN (with antioxidants – vitamins A, C, and E; folate; zinc; and copper) in women with low levels of these during preconception resulted in better serum and follicular levels and reduction of oxidative stress.[20]

Increased antioxidant intake can also help reduce the time of pregnancy. In this regard, research shows the beneficial effect of vitamin C in women of average weight (BMI <25 kg/m^2), β-carotene in overweight women (BMI $\geqslant 25$ kg/m^2), β-carotene and vitamin C in women aged <35 years, and vitamin E in women aged $\geqslant 35$ years.[21]

Another study regarding antioxidants found that supplementation of micronutrients that have antioxidant effects (e.g., vitamins B_2, B_6, C, and E; copper; manganese; zinc; selenium) in older women ($\geqslant 39$ years) before IVF cycles significantly increased the mean number of good-quality oocytes retrieved (the result of decreased oxidative stress) and the pregnancy rate of 17.7%. Multiple micronutrient supplementation can also significantly improve embryo quality in older women (>35 years) undergoing ICSI/IVF.[12]

If there is one more nutritive supplement that needs special mention, it is coenzyme Q_{10} (CoQ_{10}). This supplement has been found to:[22–24]

- Restore oocyte mitochondrial function and fertility during reproductive ageing.
- Improve ovarian response to stimulation and embryological parameters in young women with poor ovarian reserve in IVF-ICSI cycles.
- Enhance egg quality in women who have a history of infertility or previous miscarriages.

In summary, micronutrient supplementation has a small but beneficial effect on fertility in healthy and infertile women. It is not only associated with a shorter time to pregnancy but also with an increased likelihood of achieving pregnancy. Regarding the risks of preconceptional MMN supplementation, available safety data indicate that supplementation is well tolerated. However, gastrointestinal adverse events have been reported with MMN supplementation.[12] It is thus ideal for chalking out a safe, individualized treatment plan in consultation with a healthcare practitioner.

Key Takeaways

- A woman's fertility is favoured by well-balanced healthy diets such as the Mediterranean and fertility diets.
- Micronutrient supplementation has a small but beneficial effect on fertility in healthy and infertile women. It is not only associated with a shorter time to pregnancy but also with an increased likelihood of attaining pregnancy.
- Exercise and yoga can help relieve stress and improve fertility and the outcomes of assisted reproductive technology procedures.

Fertility, Diet, and Lifestyle Word Scramble

Put on your thinking cap and fetch your pen. Here's a list of words to unscramble. Something to help you remember what you read so far! 😉

VCDAOAO ____________________

ARERADITEENNM ____________________

CURIOTEINSTRMN ____________________

SHCIPNA ____________________

SXEESFDAL ____________________

EREXSIEC ____________________

SAEDNUTOOMRNTAU ____________________

CILFO DIAC ____________________

HYTHLEA ____________________

LSMGEUE ____________________

BERIF ____________________

Answers

1. AVOCADO
2. MEDITERRANEAN
3. MICRONUTRIENTS
4. SPINACH
5. FLAXSEEDS
6. EXERCISE
7. MONOUNSATURATED
8. FOLIC ACID
9. HEALTHY
10. LEGUMES
11. FIBRE

References

13. NHS. Eating a balanced diet. Available at: https://www.nhs.uk/live-well/eat-well/. Accessed on: 10 August 2019.

14. Harvard T.H. Chan School of Public Health. Healthy Eating Plate. Available at: https://www.hsph.harvard.edu/nutritionsource/healthy-eating-plate/. It was accessed on 10 August 2019.

15. Silvestris E, *et al.* Nutrition and female fertility: An interdependent correlation. *Front. Endocrinol.* 2019;10:346–358.

16. Szostak-Węgierek D. Nutrition and fertility. *Med Wieku Rozwoj.* 2011;15(4):431–436.

17. Harvard Health Publishing. Harvard Medical School. Follow The Fertility Diet? Available at: https://www.health.harvard.edu/diseases-and-conditions/follow-fertility-diet. Accessed on: 10 August 2019.

18. Academy of Nutrition and Dietetics. Eat right. Foods That Can Affect Fertility. Available at: https://www.eatright.org/health/pregnancy/fertility-and-reproduction/fertility-foods. It was accessed on 10 August 2019.

19. Shammas MA. Telomeres, lifestyle, cancer, and aging. *Curr Opin Clin Nutr Metab Care.* 2011;14(1):28–34.

20. Balan E, Decottignies A, Deldicque L. Physical activity and nutrition: Two promising strategies for telomere maintenance? *Nutrients.* 2018;10(12):1942.

21. Vidaček NS, Nanić L, Ravlić S, *et al.* Telomeres, nutrition, and longevity: Can we navigate our aging? *The Journals of Gerontology: Series A.* 2018;73(1): 39–47.

22. The Fertility Society of Australia. The role of exercise in improving fertility, quality of life, and emotional wellbeing. Available at: https://www.yourfertility.org.au/sites/default/files/2018-

08/The_role_of_exercise_in_improving_fertility.pdf. Accessed on: 8 Aug 2019.

23. Yoga for Inner Peace: A Stress-Relieving Sequence. Available at: https://www.yogajournal.com/practice/yoga-for-inner-peace-stress-relief-daily-practice-challenge#gid=ci0207569e402525bd&pid=colleen-saidman-yee-performs-easy-pose-with-forward-bend. Accessed on: 8 Aug 2019.

24. Schaefer E, Nock D. The Impact of preconceptional multiple-micronutrient supplementation on female fertility. *Clin Med Insights Womens Health.* 2019;12:1179562X19843868.

25. La Vecchia I, Paffoni A, Castiglioni M, *et al.* Folate, homocysteine and selected vitamins and minerals status in infertile women. *Eur J Contracept Reprod Health Care.* 2017;22:70–75.

26. Grajecki D, Zyriax B-C, Buhling K. The effect of micronutrient supplements on female fertility: A systematic review. *Arch Gynecol Obstet.* 2012;285:1463–1471.

27. Fung JL, Hartman TJ, Schleicher RL, *et al.* Association of vitamin D intake and serum levels with fertility: The lifestyle and fertility study results. *Fertil Steril.* 2017;108:302–311.

28. Pludowski P, Holick MF, Pilz S, *et al.* Vitamin D affects musculoskeletal health, immunity, autoimmunity, cardiovascular disease, cancer, fertility, pregnancy, dementia and mortality—A review of recent evidence. *Autoimmun Rev.* 2013;12:976–989.

29. Lerchbaum E, Obermayer-Pietsch B. Vitamin D, and fertility: A systematic review. *Eur J Endocrinol.* 2012;166:765–778.

30. Fenkci V, Fenkci S, Yilmazer M, *et al.* Decreased total antioxidant status and increased oxidative stress in women with polycystic ovary syndrome may contribute to the risk of cardiovascular disease. *Fertil Steril.* 2003;80:123–127.

31. Andrews MA, Schliep KC, Wactawski-Wende J, *et al.* Dietary factors and luteal phase deficiency in healthy eumenorrheic women. *Hum Reprod.* 2015;30:1942–1951.

32. Ozkaya MO, Naziroglu M. Multivitamin and mineral supplementation modulate oxidative stress and antioxidant vitamin levels in serum and follicular fluid of women undergoing in vitro fertilization. *Fertil Steril.* 2010;94:2465–2466.

33. Ruder EH, Hartman TJ, Reindollar RH, *et al.* Female dietary antioxidant intake and time to pregnancy among couples treated for unexplained infertility. *Fertil Steril.* 2014;101:759–766.

34. Xu Y, Nisenblat V, Lu C, *et al.* Pretreatment with coenzyme Q10 improves ovarian response and embryo quality in low-prognosis young women with decreased ovarian reserve: A randomized controlled trial. *Reprod Biol Endocrinol.* 2018;16(1):29.

35. Ben-Meir A, Burstein E, Borrego-Alvarez A, *et al.* Coenzyme Q10 restores oocyte mitochondrial function and fertility during reproductive aging. *Aging Cell.* 2015;14(5):887–895.

36. Rebecca Fett. It Starts with the Egg: How the Science of Egg Quality Can Help You Get Pregnant Naturally, Prevent Miscarriage, and Improve Your Odds of IVF. 2nd edn. Franklin Fox Publishing: New York, 2014.

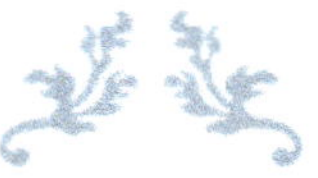

Sam owns an automotive spare parts company. Being the only son of his parents, he had an affluent lifestyle. The consequences of his affluence were obesity and excessive alcohol intake. Sam never paid heed to his lifestyle. He did very little physical activity: he spent most of his day slouched at the cash counter; his meals comprised fast foods. He rarely consumed home-cooked, fresh food.

After being married for five years, worried about not being able to have children, Sam's wife finally convinced him to meet a doctor. What he thought would be a simple visit to the doctor, turned out to be a nightmare. Little did Sam realise he had a fertility problem!

Sam's life was shattered; he was filled with remorse at having disappointed his wife. However, to his relief, the doctor assured the couple that his problem could probably be resolved if he opted to diligently change his lifestyle. Little did Sam know that his unhealthy lifestyle and diet can impact his fertility.

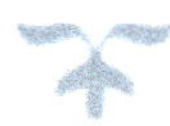

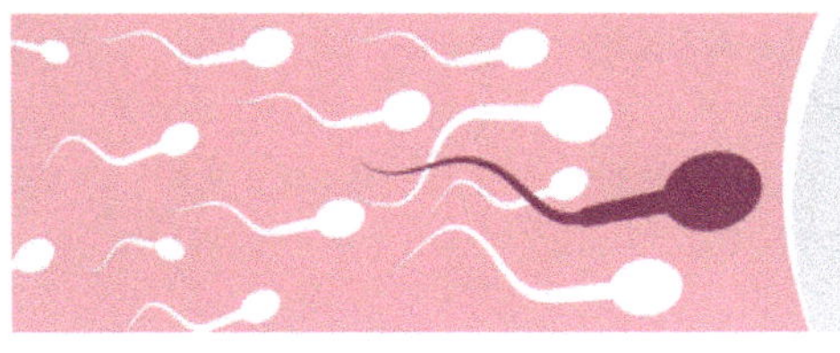

Chapter 3 Nutrition and Male Fertility

Historically, fertility issues have typically been associated with women. However, of late, many couples have come to realize that infertility may be due to problems in men. Up to 30% of fertility problems are attributable to difficulties in men.[1]

Most men are unaware that sperm quality and quantity are closely linked to male fecundity (reproductive capacity). There has been a dramatic decline in male fertility worldwide in the past few years.[1,2] The question is, why are we witnessing this trend? Evidence shows that poor nutrition and diet are among the many factors that can adversely influence male fertility.[3]

When Diet Becomes a Debacle

Unhealthy eating indeed affects males of reproductive age. Changes in dietary patterns, such as a high intake of saturated fatty acids, trans fats, and sodium and a low intake of fruits and vegetables (both of which are rich in antioxidants and flavonoids), could be a few among the many triggers for male infertility.[4] Rapid urbanization has paved the way for establishing a non-traditional, "fast food" culture. These days, most people consume processed

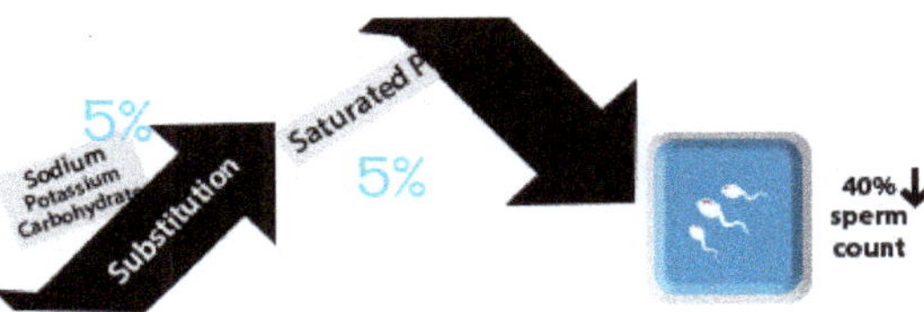

meat, soya foods, potatoes, full-fat dairy products, coffee, alcohol, sugar-sweetened beverages, and sweets because of the palatability, affordability, variety, and easy availability associated with these foods. Early adoption of fast food culture can harm male fertility.[5]

Common nutrition-related factors resulting in male infertility

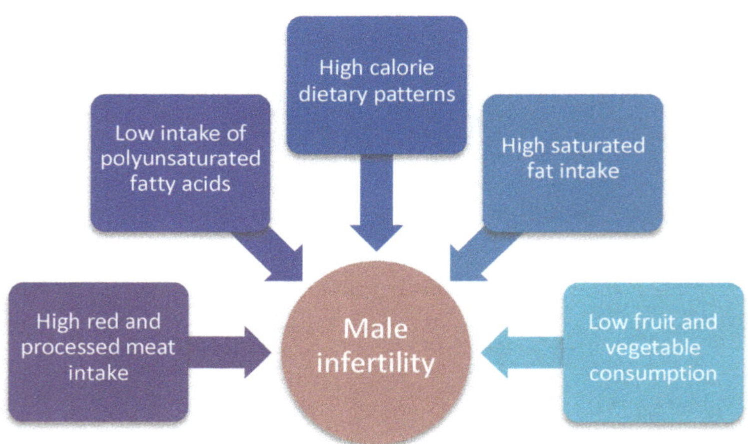

You Are What You Eat

Eating habits – more specifically, the consumption pattern of both macro and micro-nutrients – influence reproductive function. For example, a 5% increase in total energy from fat can drop sperm counts by 18%.[6]

Unhealthy dietary patterns, which typically involve the frequent consumption of sweets, snacks, processed meat, animal fat, red meat, refined grain products, potatoes, and dairy products, increase the risk of abnormal sperm motility and morphology – in addition to reducing sperm motility (asthenozoospermia) and concentration.[7]

Carbohydrates

Men with a sweet tooth are not only at risk for obesity or metabolic disorders like cardiac diseases and diabetes but also infertility! High intake of sugar-laden snacks and beverages is inversely linked to sperm counts and sperm motility, especially among young, healthy men. This can be attributed to a phenomenon called insulin resistance.[8]

Insulin is a hormone that regulates blood sugar levels in the body, and insulin resistance is a condition wherein the body does not heed the signal insulin is trying to send out. Insulin resistance increases oxidative stress (an imbalance between free radicals and antioxidants). Oxidative stress, in turn, adversely impacts sperm motility.[8]

Mounting evidence highlights that increased intake of soft drinks (>14´0.5 L bottles/week) and/or caffeine (>800 mg/day) could reduce sperm concentration and sperm counts.[8]

Proteins

Soya protein is considered an ideal source of protein. The downside of soya protein is high levels of isoflavones, which adversely affect male sperm parameters. While more research is required on these aspects,

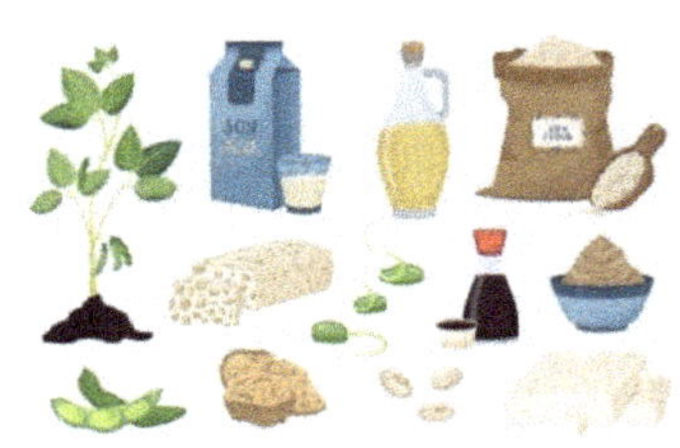

some studies have demonstrated that, compared to infertile men who did not consume soya foods, the sperm concentration was significantly lower by 41 million sperm per mL among infertile men who consumed a high quantity of soya.[6]

Soya is a meat analogue for burgers, sausages, bacon, and hot dogs. Soya or soya sauce is used in various foods, including salad dressings, soups, beverage powders, and cheeses.[6]

Consuming whole-fat dairy products decreases sperm motility and negatively alters sperm morphology.[3] Oligoasthenoteratospermia is a reduction in the motility and number of spermatozoa and a change in their morphology. Studies have reported that men with oligoasthenoteratospermia typically have a higher intake of full-fat dairy products (yogurt, whole milk, cheese, and semi-skimmed milk) and lower skimmed milk intake than men with normal sperm. The risk of asthenozoospermia is also marginally higher with a greater intake of total dairy products and significantly lower with a greater intake of skimmed milk.[9]

Fats

While your favorite steak is just a call away, you may want to understand why consuming processed meat isn't a great idea. Animal products contribute to a deterioration in sperm quality: the saturated fatty acids and natural trans fatty acids in animal-based products negatively influence sperm count, concentration, and testicular metabolism.[4,6] Further, if the diet has a higher content of processed meat, such as sausages, there is an increased likelihood of poor semen quality.[6]

Omega-3 polyunsaturated fatty acids (a type of polyunsaturated fatty acid, PUFA) have a role in male fertility disorders. Docosahexaenoic acid (DHA; omega-3 fatty acid) levels are lower in the spermatozoa of men with asthenozoospermia than in men without asthenozoospermia. The blood and spermatozoa of fertile men have higher concentrations of omega-3-PUFAs compared to men with idiopathic (a medical condition that has no known cause) infertility.[6]

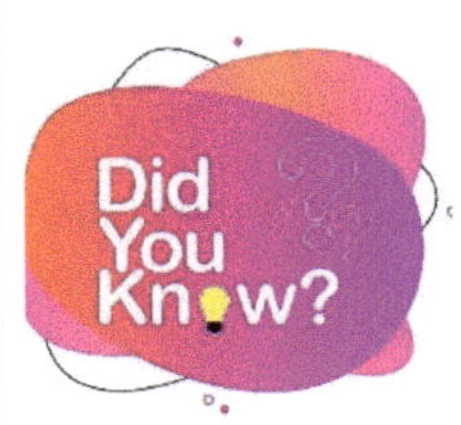

Pesticides may be the pesty little monsters messing with your fertility! [9,10]

Men with an increased intake of high-pesticide–residue fruit and vegetables (≥1.5 servings/day) have been shown to have 49% lower total sperm counts and 32% lower morphologically normal sperm compared to men with lower intake (<0.5 servings/day) of such fruit and vegetables. Low-to-moderate-pesticide—residue fruit and vegetable intake has been linked to a higher percentage of morphologically normal sperm.

While fruits and vegetables are universally recommended as essential components of a healthy diet, they are also the primary sources of pesticide residue. Here are a few tips to reduce the pesticide residue of the food you eat:

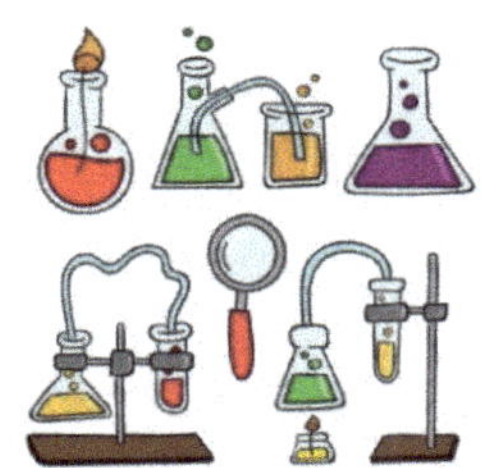

- ✓ Thoroughly wash all produce. Don't forget the organic ones and even those that must be peeled.

- ✓ Ensure you wash all produce under running water rather than merely soaking or dunking it in water.
- ✓ Firm fruits and vegetables such as root vegetables can be scrubbed.
- ✓ Dry out produce with a clean cloth towel if possible.
- ✓ Discard the outer layer of leafy vegetables like lettuce and cabbage.
- ✓ Make sure to peel fruits and vegetables whenever possible.

Not only fruits and vegetables but even meat can carry pesticides. Here's a bonus tip – trim fat and skin from meat, poultry, and fish to minimize exposure to pesticide residue.

Body Weight Counts

Obese men are more likely to experience infertility. Moreover, clinical pregnancy and live birth rates per assisted reproduction cycle are reduced in obese men. Obesity in males adversely impacts spermatogenesis, sperm count (oligozoospermia and azoospermia), and, most importantly, sperm DNA integrity, a crucial element for a healthy pregnancy.[11]

Meal-skipping is one of the most frequently used but least effective weight-control methods. Many people are not aware that inappropriate dietary habits, such as skipping meals or false dieting, could be responsible for male infertility.[4]

Non-nutritive Substances

Psssstttt.......
Parenting begins before conception!

Paternal obesity has been shown to affect embryo development, pregnancy outcomes, and body fat in offspring.[12–14] Not just the embryo, even the offspring is affected. While a low-protein paternal diet changes lipid and cholesterol metabolism in offspring, a high-fat paternal diet leads to beta-cell dysfunction and consequently diabetes in daughters.[14,15] While we await more solid evidence from human studies, research in rat models has shed some light on this subject.

It has been said that the live birth rate of couples among whom the male partner has a caffeine intake of ≥272 mg/day is approximately three times lower compared to couples among whom the male partner has a caffeine intake of <99 mg/day.[3]

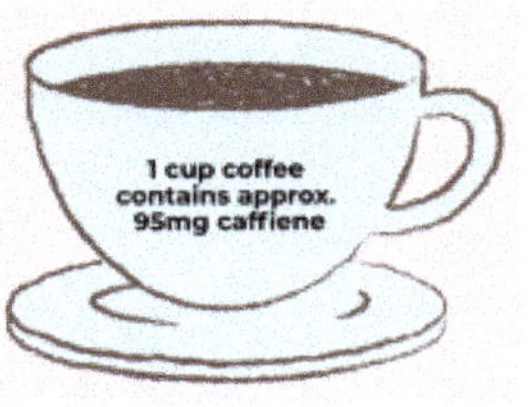

Alcohol consumption has been related to low sperm volume and high sperm DNA fragmentation. Infertile men who drink 2–3 units of alcoholic beverages per day have a much lower semen quality compared with occasional drinkers (<3 units per week). Alcohol consumption also increases the number of morphologically abnormal sperms.[3]

Last but not least, smoking. Smoking not only has unfavorable effects on male semen parameters; it also reportedly reduces the success of assisted reproduction techniques, such as *in vitro* fertilization (IVF) and intracytoplasmic sperm injection (ICSI).[16]

Key Takeaways

- Poor diet and lifestyle adversely impact male fertility.
- Several foods and specific nutrients play a role in male fertility.
- Unhealthy dietary patterns, which typically involve frequent consumption of sweets, snacks, processed meat, animal fat, red meat, refined grain products, potatoes, and dairy products, can affect fertility.
- Obese men are more likely to experience infertility. Paternal obesity has been shown to affect embryo development, pregnancy outcomes, and body fat in offspring.

Nutrition and Male Fertility - Match the Following

Match the following in List A with that in List B in the correct order.

Sl no.	**A**	**B**
1	Pesticide residues	Soya and soya products
2	Saturated fatty acids and natural trans fatty acids	Omega-3 fats
3	Isoflavones	Fruits and vegetables
4	Docosahexaenoic acid	Paternal obesity
5	Impaired embryo development and pregnancy outcomes	Animal products

Answers

A	**B**
Pesticide residues	Fruits and vegetables
Saturated fatty acids and natural trans fatty acids	Animal products
Isoflavones	Soya and soya products
Docosahexaenoic acid	Omega-3 fats

Impaired embryo development and pregnancy outcomes	Paternal obesity

References

1. Levine H, Jorgensen N, Martino-Andrade A, *et al.* Temporal trends in sperm count: A systematic review and meta-regression analysis. *Hum Reprod Update.* 2017;23(6):646–659.

2. Ricci E, Al-Beitawi S, Cipriani S, *et al.* Dietary habits and semen parameters: A systematic narrative review. *Andrology.* 2018;6:104–116.

3. Çekici H. Current nutritional factors are affecting fertility and infertility. *Ann Clin Lab Res.* 2018;6(1):225.

4. Giahi L, Mohammadmoradi S, Javidan A, *et al.* Nutritional modifications in male infertility: A systematic review covering two decades.*Nutr Rev.* 2016;74(2):118–130.

5. Salas-Huetos A, Bulló M, Salas-Salvadó J. Dietary patterns, foods and nutrients in male fertility parameters and fecundability: A systematic review of observational studies. *Hum Reprod Update.* 2017;23(4):371–389.

6. Hosseini B, Djafarian K. Dietary nutrients and male infertility: Review of current evidence. *GMJ.* 2015;4(4):123–129.

7. Danielewicz A, Przybyłowicz KE, Przybyłowicz M. Dietary patterns and poor semen quality risk in men: A cross-sectional study. *Nutrients.* 2018;10(9):1162.

8. Liu CY, Chou YC, Chao JC, *et al.* The association between dietary patterns and semen quality in a general Asian population of 7282 males. *PLoS One.* 2015;10(7):e0134224.

9. Nassan FL, Chavarro JE, Tanrikut C. Diet, and men's fertility: Does diet affect sperm quality? *Fertil Steril.* 2018;110(4):570–577.
10. National Pesticide Information Center. Minimizing Pesticide Residues in Food. Available at: http://npic.orst.edu/health/foodprac.html. Accessed on 20 August 2019.
11. Roger Hart and Tamara Hunter (December 31st, 2018). Reproductive Consequences of Obesity [Online First], IntechOpen, DOI: 10.5772/intechopen.80897. Available from: https://www.intechopen.com/online-first/reproductive-consequences-of-obesity. It was accessed on 20 August 2019.
12. Dodd JM, Du Plessis LE, Deussen AR, *et al.* Paternal obesity modifies the effect of an antenatal lifestyle intervention in women who are overweight or obese on newborn anthropometry. *Sci Rep.* 2017;7(1):1557.
13. Binder NK, Hannan NJ, Gardner DK. Paternal diet-induced obesity retards early mouse embryo development, mitochondrial activity, and pregnancy health. *PLoS One.* 2012;7(12):e52304.
14. Lane M, Robker RL, Robertson SA. Parenting from before conception. *Science.* 2014:756–760.
15. Ng SF, Lin RC, Laybutt DR, *et al.* Chronic high-fat diet in fathers programs β-cell dysfunction in female rat offspring. *Nature.* 2010;467(7318):963–966.
16. Kovac JR, Khanna A, Lipshultz LI. The effects of cigarette smoking on male fertility. *Postgrad Med.* 2015;127(3):338–341.

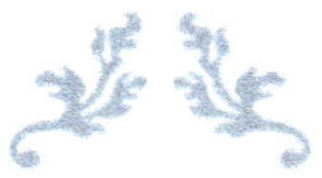

The food you eat can be either the safest and most powerful form of medicine or the slowest form of poison.

–Ann Wigmore

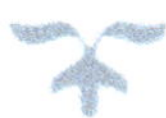

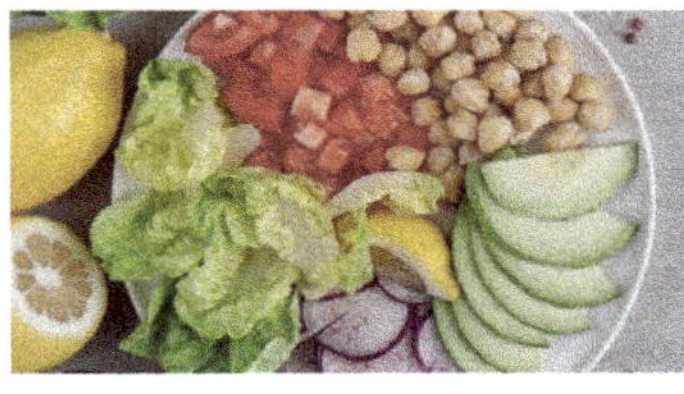

Chapter 4 Male Fertility: Diet and Lifestyle

We've caught a glimpse of how a poor diet hampers fertility; now, let's learn how good food can boost the chances of paternity.

It All Starts With Food

Special attention to certain foods and food groups can improve fertility.

Every sperm is encapsulated within a cell membrane. The cell membrane is critical in fertilization and is highly important for proper sperm function. Docosahexaenoic acid (DHA, a type of omega-3 polyunsaturated fat) is an integral element of the cell membrane. Optimal sperm membrane DHA content is linked to higher sperm motility and normal sperm morphology and concentration.[1] Fish, seafood, and shellfish potentially benefit sperm parameters due to their high omega-3 content.[2] Studies have demonstrated that in couples trying to conceive, higher fish intake by men cuts down the risk of infertility (better sperm count and normal sperm morphology) and shortens the time taken to conceive.[1]

But what if you're not a fan of seafood? Worry not; walnuts are yet another rich source of omega-3 fats. Walnut supplementation of 75 g/day for 12 weeks in young, healthy men has boosted sperm vitality, motility, and morphology.[1] Eicosapentaenoic acid

(EPA; another type of omega-3 polyunsaturated fat) and DHA also offer anti-inflammatory and antioxidant benefits.[2]

Fruits, vegetables, legumes, and whole cereals are beneficial. Why, what do they have in common? If you guessed fibre, you are right! Fibre consumption lowers plasma estrogen levels in males, essential for normal fertility. Besides, fruits and vegetables contain antioxidants (vitamins A and C, β-carotene, polyphenols, other phytochemicals, potassium, magnesium) and folate. Antioxidants scavenge reactive oxygen species (ROS) and folate, which supports deoxyribonucleic acid (DNA) synthesis, a vital part of spermatogenesis.[2]

> Reactive oxygen species negatively affect sperm DNA and, therefore, sperm motility, vitality, and concentration. Reactive oxygen species also leads to miscarriage and the developmental abnormalities in offspring.[2]

Like the fertility diet for women, low-fat, skimmed milk benefits men's fertility. Skimmed milk is associated with higher peripheral concentrations of insulin-like growth factor 1 (IGF-1) and insulin, necessary for spermatogenesis.[1,2]

Diet That Makes a Difference

The Mediterranean diet (MedDiet) should be your go-to diet. It not only features all the foods beneficial for fertility (seafood, poultry, whole grains, legumes, skimmed milk, fruits, and vegetables) but also helps consume the right quantities. Owing to

Take a sneak peek at the MedDiet pyramid in Chapter 2.

its nutritional profile – high omega-3 fat, antioxidant, and vitamin content and low saturated fat and trans-fat content – the MedDiet has been consistently associated with better semen parameters. Men adhering to this diet benefit from higher sperm concentrations and total sperm count, as well as sperm motility. Furthermore, this healthy diet pattern is associated with lower sperm DNA fragmentation. No doubt the MedDiet positively impacts male reproductive potential.[1,2]

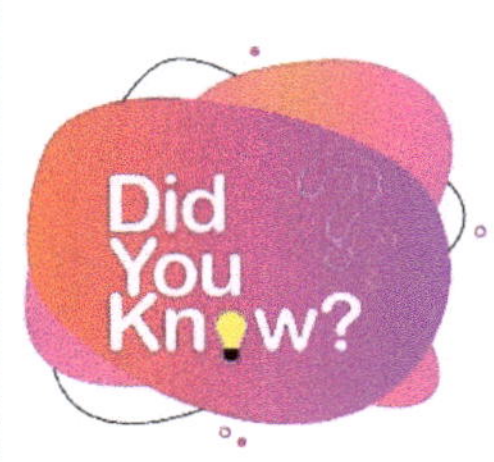

Keto Diet Is a Fad Diet, Not a Fab Diet for Weight Loss[3,4]

Lately, the keto diet has received immense limelight; however, it is not something new. Initially designed for patients with epilepsy, the ketogenic diet requires one to forgo nearly all carbohydrates, avoid excess protein, and consume high levels of fat, resulting in the production of ketones (giving the diet its name). The diet features plenty of eggs, processed meat, sausage, cheese, fish, nuts, butter, oils, seeds, and fibrous vegetables. Surprisingly, the diet isn't famous for its benefits for epilepsy but rather for weight loss.

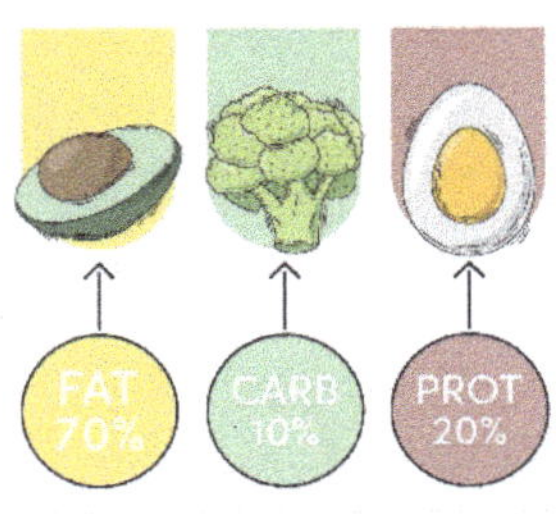

Keto Diet for Weight Loss: Can We Count on It?

Essentially, any diet that results in weight loss is linked to reduced calorie intake. The ketogenic diet, when used for weight loss, is no different. However, the question remains: is it sustainable, and does it promote health in the long run? Because, after all, weight loss must be long-lasting and healthy.

In reality, many people following this diet overeat protein and poor-quality fats from processed food with very few fruits and vegetables. Eating patterns tend to lean towards a heavy intake of red meat and other fatty, processed, and salty foods that are notoriously unhealthy. Moreover, a low-carbohydrate diet is linked to increased all-cause mortality. Not to forget, whole grains, fruits, and legumes are health-promoting foods, so letting them go may not be the best idea.

The keto diet is associated with several adverse effects, ranging from the keto flu, fatigue, and weakness to gastrointestinal disturbances. Rarely, fatal cardiac arrhythmias from selenium deficiency may occur. Some of the other side effects are nephrolithiasis, constipation, halitosis, muscle cramps, headaches, diarrhea, bone fractures, pancreatitis, and multiple vitamin and mineral deficiencies.

The latest article published in the renowned Journal of the American Medical Association states, "The evidence supporting the use of ketogenic diet for the dietary treatment of obesity is currently limited, and the diet's potential risks are real."

Last but not least, owing to its restrictions, the diet is rigid to stick to, and people

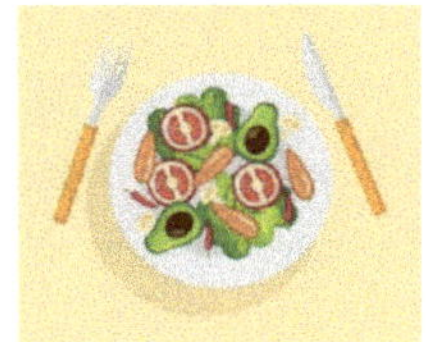

cannot follow this eating pattern over a long period. Remember that "yo-yo diets" that lead to rapid weight loss fluctuation are linked with increased mortality; rather than following the next popular diet that would last only a few weeks or months, embrace a balanced, healthy, sustainable diet change over the long term.

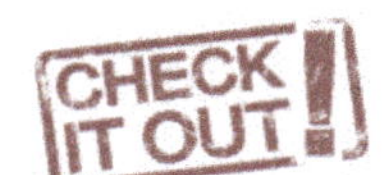

Diet and exercise go hand in hand in weight loss and good health. Flip back to Chapter 2 for more information on weight loss.

Supplementation to Boost Chances of Paternity

Mounting evidence shows that oxidative stress plays a vital role in male infertility. Reactive oxygen species, the main culprit for oxidative stress, have been shown to impair sperm function and motility and damage the sperm membrane and DNA.[5,6]

ThinkByte

Both lack of exercise and intensive exercise generate high levels of oxidative stress.[7]

Get to know more about the right amount of exercise in Chapter 2.

Antioxidants keep a check on ROS and, thereby, reduce oxidative stress. In the event of lower levels of antioxidants, the balance tilts towards a higher level of seminal oxidative stress and can consequently lead to infertility. In this milieu, oral antioxidant therapy could help combat seminal ROS and restore the redox balance.[5,6]

Improvements in the total antioxidant capacity of seminal fluids seem to contribute to improving key semen parameters such as sperm morphology and motility. Vitamin E (400 mg), vitamin C (500–1000 mg), co-enzyme Q_{10} (CoQ_{10}; 100–300 mg), zinc (25–400 mg), selenium (200 mg), and folic acid (0.5 mg) are the most commonly used antioxidant supplements. The mechanism by which antioxidants increase sperm concentration might be either due to the suppression of ROS-induced sperm damage or through some other unknown mechanism.[5,6]

Antioxidant	Action	Food sources
Vitamin C	Neutralizes free radicals	Citrus fruits, bell peppers, berries
Vitamin E	Inhibits free radical induced damage to cell membranes	Wheat germ, cereals/grains, egg, fruits and vegetables
Folate (Folic acid)	Scavenges free radicals; involved in DNA synthesis	Dark green leafy vegetables, beans, eggs
Selenium	Enhancement of enzymatic antioxidant activities	Brazilian nuts, cereals, seafood, eggs
Zinc	DNA synthesis; inhibits NADPH oxidase	Wheat, seeds (sunflower, sesame, pumpkin)
CoQ_{10}	Stabilize and protect the cell membrane from oxidative stress	Mackerel, sardines, whole grain, rice bran, soybeans, nuts, vegetables

Since a sperm takes 72 days to mature, it is prudent to give antioxidant supplements for a minimum of three months to men experiencing high levels of oxidative stress.[5]

Three months' treatment with vitamins A, E, and C and selenium significantly increases sperm motility. Men with asthenoteratozoospermia can reap significant benefits from a combination of antioxidants that includes beta-glucan, fermented papaya, lactoferrin, vitamin C, and vitamin E, in terms of a substantial improvement in the percentage of morphologically normal sperm cells and progressive sperm motility.[5]

Daily supplementation of vitamin C in infertile men with idiopathic (medical condition that has no known cause) oligozoospermia has been found to significantly increase sperm motility count, as well as the percentage of normal spermatozoa.[5]

Selenium also impacts sperm morphology in the epididymis. Sperms can be spared from oxidative damage if selenium is provided as selenoproteins. Selenium and vitamin E supplementation for over three months helps men improve their sperm parameters, especially those with oligoasthenoteratozoospermia, for unknown reasons. Further, the supplementation also helped their spouses (10.8%) conceive spontaneously.[5,8]

Zinc is a vital component for testicular development, steroidogenesis, and the formation and maturation of spermatozoa.[5] Several studies have highlighted improvement in sperm concentration, progressive motility, sperm integrity, and pregnancy rates in subfertile men after zinc supplementation.[9]

Zinc and folic acid are essential for DNA synthesis in sperms. Daily 5 mg folic acid supplementation and 66 mg zinc in subfertile men have demonstrated a staggering 74% increase in total average sperm count.[9]

Oral supplementation of 60 mg CoQ_{10} in infertile men has shown an enhanced fertilization rate, although it was not associated with improved semen parameters.[9] Research has unearthed that omega-3 supplementation for more than four weeks improves sperm analysis results.[10]

In summary, while more research is warranted on the role of supplementation in infertility, supplementation of certain nutrients has been shown to have a small but beneficial effect on fertility in men. Remember, choosing a safe, individualized treatment plan is always best in consultation with a healthcare practitioner.

Key Takeaways

- Male fertility is improved by consuming well-balanced healthy diets such as the Mediterranean diet.
- Avoiding fad diets for weight loss and opting for a healthy diet and adequate exercise is recommended.
- Supplementation of certain nutrients has a small but beneficial effect on fertility in men.

Crossword Puzzle on Diet and Lifestyle for Men's Fertility

Solving crossword puzzles is like mental yoga — both challenging and relaxing at the same time. Solve this crossword grid and get your dose of mental yoga today.

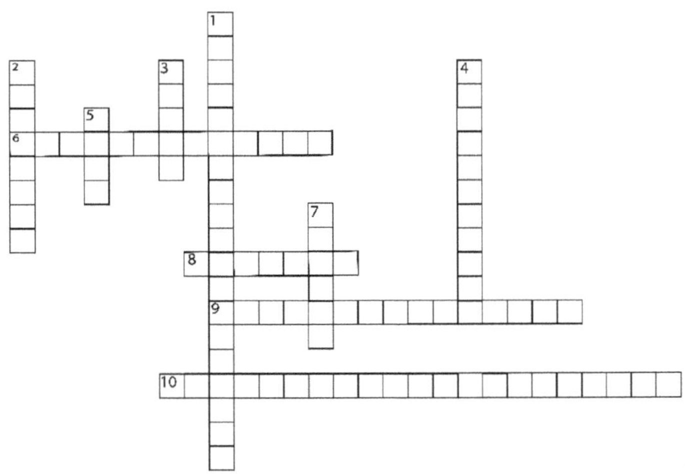

ACROSS

6 A diet that can boost the chances of paternity.

8 It's a trending fad diet.

9 Both lack of exercise and intensive levels of exercise generate high levels of:

10 ____________ adversely impacts several aspects of the sperm. It also leads to miscarriage and developmental abnormalities in the offspring.

DOWN

1 A type of omega-3 fat that is beneficial for male fertility.

2 A type of milk that can help boost male fertility.

3 A nutrient common to fruits, vegetables, legumes, and whole cereals.

4 Vitamin E, vitamin C, co-enzyme Q_{10}, zinc, and selenium are commonly used ________ supplements for improving fertility in men.

5 Folic acid and _____ are essential for DNA synthesis in sperms.

7 Fish, seafood, and shellfish are excellent sources of:

Answers

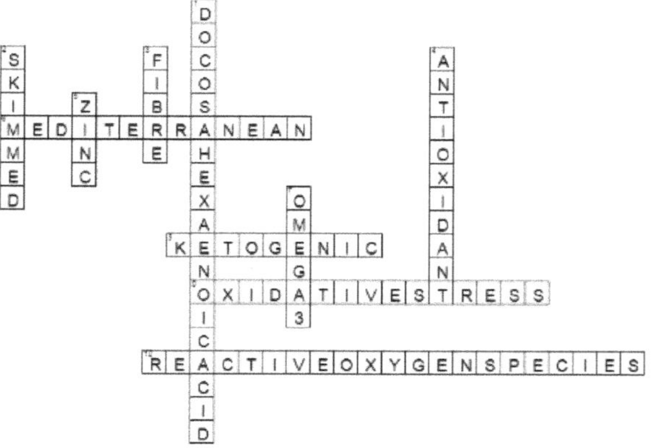

References

37. Nassan FL, Chavarro JE, Tanrikut C. Diet, and men's fertility: Does diet affect sperm quality? *Fertil Steril.* 2018;110(4):570–577.

38. Salas-Huetos A, Bulló M, Salas-Salvadó J. Dietary patterns, foods and nutrients in male fertility parameters and fecundability: A systematic review of observational studies. *Human Reproduction Update.* 2017;23(4):371–389.

39. Joshi S, Ostfeld RJ, McMacken. The ketogenic diet for obesity and diabetes—Enthusiasm outpaces evidence. *JAMA Intern Med.* Online. 2019.

40. Harvard Health Publishing. Ketogenic diet: Is the ultimate low-carb diet good for you? Available at: https://www.health.harvard.edu/blog/ketogenic-diet-is-the-ultimate-low-carb-diet-good-for-you-2017072712089. Accessed on: 8 August 2019.

41. Alahmar AT. The effects of oral antioxidants on the semen of men with idiopathic oligoasthenoteratozoospermia. *Clin Exp Reprod Med.* 2018;45(2):57–66.

42. Majzoub A, Agarwal A. Systematic review of antioxidant types and doses in male infertility: Benefits on semen parameters, advanced sperm function, assisted reproduction and live-birth rate. *Arab J Urology.* 2018;16(1):113–124.

43. Kefer JC, Agarwal A, Sabanegh E. Role of antioxidants in treating male infertility. *Int J Urol.* 2009;16:449–457

44. Robbins WA, Xun L, FitzGerald LZ, *et al.* Walnuts improve semen quality in men consuming a western-style diet: Randomized control dietary intervention trial. *Biol Reprod.* 2012;87(4)101:1–8.

45. Mora-Esteves C, Shin D. Nutrient supplementation: Improving male fertility fourfold. *Semin Reprod Med.* 2013;31:293–300.

46. Peres HA, Freitas Foss MC, *et al.* An update- The role of nutrients crucial in couples' infertility- New insights for the effects of iodine, selenium, omega three fatty acids, and magnesium. *J Nutrition Health Food Sci.* 2017;5(7):1–6.

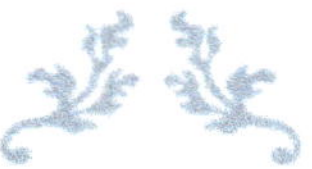

"Go on! Help yourself! You're eating for two now!" was a common remark Susan heard once she had announced that she was pregnant. Be it at home, office, or social gatherings, people never failed to push her to eat more, and it would make her cringe. Susan wanted to make sure she was eating enough for the baby's growth; at the same time, she remembered how her friend had ended up with several complications after packing on too many pounds during her pregnancy. Susan was keen on striking a balance.

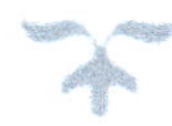

Chapter 5 Nutrition for a Healthy Pregnancy

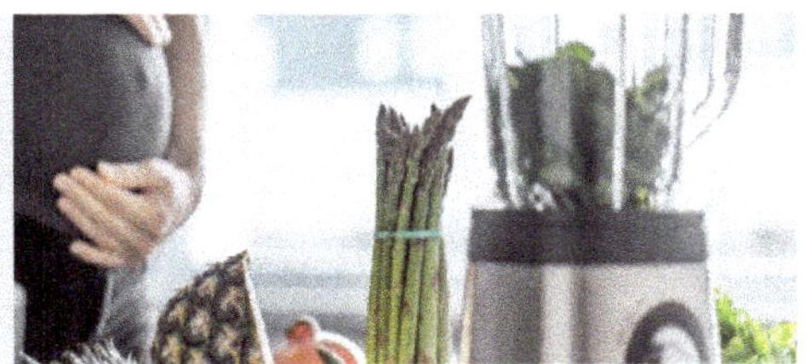

The perception that a pregnant woman should eat for two people, apart from being erroneous, can sometimes lead to overeating or the consumption of the wrong foods. Then, what is the ideal amount to consume during pregnancy, and what are the suitable types of food to eat?

Piling on the Right Number of Pounds

A mother's optimal weight gain during pregnancy is essential to support and nurture herself and the growing fetus.[1] However, excessive weight gain during pregnancy has multifaceted consequences:[2]

Read more on how weight gain during pregnancy can affect the mother's as well as the child's long-term health in Chapter 11.

- ✗ Poor pregnancy outcomes for the mother and the baby
- ✗ Increased risk of postpartum weight retention and subsequent obesity in mothers
- ✗ Large-for-gestational–age babies with excess weight during infancy

What Is the Ideal Weight Gain During Pregnancy?

Weight gain goals are in accordance with prepregnancy nutritional status and body mass index (BMI).[3,4]

How do you calculate your BMI?
BMI is a measure of body weight based on your height and weight.

BMI Formula:

$$BMI = \frac{Weight\ (kg)}{(Height\ (m))^2} \quad or \quad BMI = \frac{Weight\ (lb)}{(Height\ (in))^2} \times 70$$

If before pregnancy, you were…	You should gain…	
Underweight BMI <18.5 kg/m^2	28–40 lb	(12.5–18 kg)
Normal weight BMI 18.5–24.9 kg/m^2	25–35 lb	(11.5–16 kg)
Overweight BMI 25.0–29.9 kg/m^2	15–25 lb	(7–11.5 kg)
Obese BMI ≥30.0 kg/m^2	11–20 lb	(5–9 kg)

And if you are pregnant with twins…

If before pregnancy, you were…	You should gain…	
Underweight BMI <18.5 kg/m^2	50–62 lb*	(22–28 kg)
Normal Weight BMI 18.5–24.9 kg/m^2	37–54 lb	(16.5–24 kg)

If before pregnancy, you were...	You should gain...	
Overweight BMI 25.0–29.9 kg/m^2	31–50 lb	(14–22 kg)
Obese BMI ≥30.0 kg/m^2	25–42 lb	(11.5–19 kg)

*All recommendations are from the Institute of Medicine, except for underweight women with twins. Source: Luke B, *et al. J Reprod Med.* 2003;48:217–24.

How Fast Should the Weight Gain Be? [3]

If before pregnancy, you were...	Your weekly weight gain during the 2nd and 3rd trimesters# should be...	
Underweight BMI <18.5 kg/m^2	1–1.3 lb*	(0.44–0.58 kg)
Normal Weight BMI 18.5–24.9 kg/m^2	0.8–1 lb	(0.35–0.50 kg)
Overweight BMI 25.0–29.9 kg/m^2	0.5–0.7 lb	(0.23–0.33 kg)
Obese BMI ≤30.0 kg/m^2	0.4–0.6 lb	(0.17–0.27 kg)

#Calculations assume a 0.5–2 kg (1.1–4.4 lb) weight gain in the first trimester.

Constituents of Gestational Weight Gain

A developing baby is called a fetus. The placenta is a flat, circular organ that develops in the uterus and nourishes the growing fetus through the umbilical cord (the tube-like structure that connects the mother and the fetus). Pregnancy is associated with the growth of maternal, placental, and foetal components and gestational weight gain. The illustration below shows the various components of weight gain during pregnancy.[3]

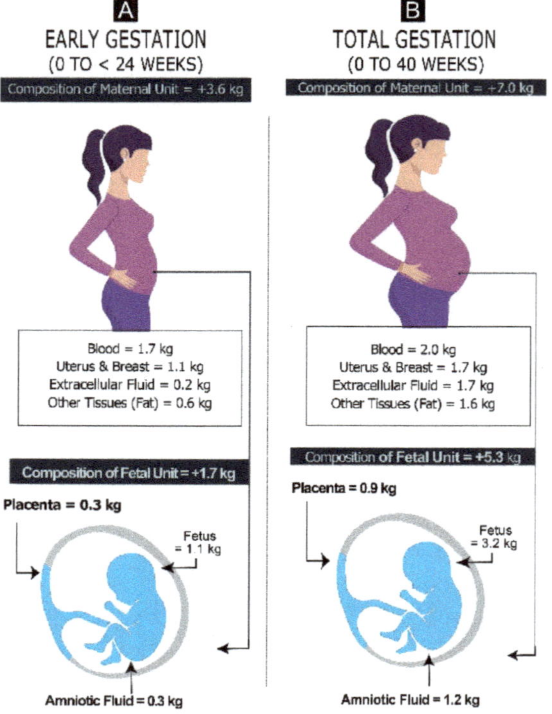

Adapted from: Carol J. Lammi-Keefe. Handbook of Nutrition and Pregnancy. 2nd edn. Humana Press: New Jersey, 2018.

Nutritional Demands During Pregnancy

Undoubtedly, foetal growth and pregnancy demand additional nutrients. As per the Food and Nutrition Board (Institute of Medicine), the recommended dietary intake for pregnant women of various age groups is detailed below.[5,6] While this can function as an essential guide, a personalized diet plan is a must. Healthcare providers and qualified dieticians/nutritionists can determine the best diet plan.

NUTRIENT	AGE 18 YEARS OR UNDER	AGES 19–30 YEARS	AGES 31–50 YEARS
Energy	1st tri = +0 kcal/d	1st tri = +0 kcal/d	1st tri = +0 kcal/d
	2nd tri = +340 kcal/d	2nd tri = +340 kcal/d	2nd tri = +340 kcal/d
	3rd tri = +452 kcal/d	3rd tri = +452 kcal/d	3rd tri = +452 kcal/d
Protein	71 g/d	71 g/d	71 g/d
Calcium	1300 mg/d	1000 mg/d	1000 mg/d
Iron	27 mg/d	27 mg/d	27 mg/d
Folate	600 μg/d	600 μg/d	600 μg/d
Phosphorus	1250 mg/d	700 mg/d	700 mg/d
Vitamin A	750 μg	770 μg	770 μg
Vitamin C	80 mg/d	85 mg/d	85 mg/d
Thiamin	1.4 mg/d	1.4 mg/d	1.4 mg/d
Riboflavin	1.4 mg/d	1.4 mg/d	1.4 mg/d
Niacin	18 mg/d	18 mg/d	18 mg/d

Adapted from Sylvia Escott-Stump. Nutrition and Diagnosis-related Care. Edition 8. Wolters Kluwer.

Here are a few tips and tricks to ensure optimal nutrition during pregnancy:[5]

- The diet and supplements should provide 27 mg of iron (ferrous form).
- Increase zinc intake by 5 mg. Milk and meat are good sources of zinc.
- Avoid excessive intake of vitamin A through supplements.
- Pregnant women need 250 μg of iodine/day; use iodized salt.
- Magnesium plays a role in preventing or correcting high blood pressure disorders. To consume sufficient magnesium, Include whole grains, nuts, black beans, green vegetables, and seafood.
- Incorporate fish and seafood (like tuna and salmon) twice weekly to ensure adequate docosahexaenoic acid (DHA) intake, which promotes brain growth and cognition.
- Always choose whole fruit over fruit juice for better fiber and antioxidant intake.
- Avoid alcohol, tobacco, cocaine, and marijuana, as they lead to decreased body weight and malformations in the offspring.
- Limit caffeine consumption to less than 200 mg/day (equivalent to two cups of coffee). And remember that caffeine is present not only in coffee but also in tea, cola, and chocolate.

Most often, pregnant women must deal with pregnancy-related symptoms like morning sickness, constipation, etc. Here are a few tips to tackle these symptoms:[5,6]

Situation	Nutrition Tips
Hyperemesis (excessive vomiting)	• Consider the intake of liquids between meals • Extra intake of B-complex vitamins, vitamin C, and limited fat intake may be beneficial.
Morning sickness (nausea and vomiting of pregnancy)	• Small, frequent meals consumed separately from fluids • Dine in a well-ventilated area, free from odors. • Eat and drink slowly, and rest after meals. • High-protein snacks (cheese/lean meat) can help. • Avoid lying down immediately after meals. • Avoid forcefully eating, skipping meals, and consuming large meals. • Avoid extremely sweet, spicy, high-fat foods and intense aromas. • Suck on ice chips and frozen fruits. • Eat dry crackers in the morning. • Ensure good rehydration.
Heartburn	• Small, frequent meals
Constipation and haemorrhoids	• Increase consumption of fibre (fruits and vegetables) and fluids • Dried fruits, especially prunes and figs, may help.

Supplementation During Pregnancy

Apart from a good dietary intake, women may require extra help of certain vital nutrients as the foetus is rapidly growing.

Folic acid: Pregnant women require at least 600 µg of folic acid daily. Since it is difficult to attain the recommended target through food alone, a daily vitamin supplement that contains folic acid is advisable.[7]

Iron: The body requires iron to produce red blood cells, which carry oxygen to all the organs and tissues in the body. During pregnancy, women require extra iron – about double the amount of iron that nonpregnant women need. The additional iron fuels the production of more blood to supply oxygen to the growing foetus. The daily recommended dose of iron during pregnancy is 27 mg, found in most prenatal vitamin supplements.[7]

> Make sure to also consume iron-rich foods such as lean red meat, poultry, fish, dried beans and peas, iron-fortified cereals, and prune juice.[7]
>
> Always remember to pair iron-rich foods with vitamin C-rich foods, such as citrus fruits and tomatoes, for better absorption of iron.[7]

Vitamin D: Vitamin D works with calcium to help the foetus's bones and teeth develop.[7] Vitamin D is found in fortified milk, juice, eggs, and fish such as salmon. The skin also produces vitamin D in the presence of sunlight. If vitamin D deficiency is discovered during pregnancy, supplements (1000–2000 international units per day) are required.[8]

Psssstttt.......

Are you using a sunscreen with sun protection factor (SPF) of 8 or more? Think twice! Such topical sunscreens block the ultraviolet (UV) rays of sunlight that are necessary for our skin to produce vitamin D. Not just that, with most of us adopting an indoor lifestyle, our exposure to sunlight is very limited.[9–11]

Pollution and smog can cut off UV rays. Did you know, people with dark skin absorb less UV rays than light-skinned people? And if you're glad that your office desk is next to a window and you sunbathe every day, don't count on making any vitamin D! Because ultraviolet B (UVB) rays (the ones your body needs to make vitamin D) can't get through the glass![9–11]

To Eat or Not to Eat?: Food Taboos During Pregnancy

Worldwide, women are often bombarded with food restrictions during pregnancy (and lactation). Food taboos and myths can often result in the restriction of foods such as meat, fruits, and vegetables during pregnancy. This can be detrimental for both the mother and the baby, since vital nutrients such as protein, vitamins, and minerals may be missed. Have a look at the food taboos and myths from around the world.[12–14]

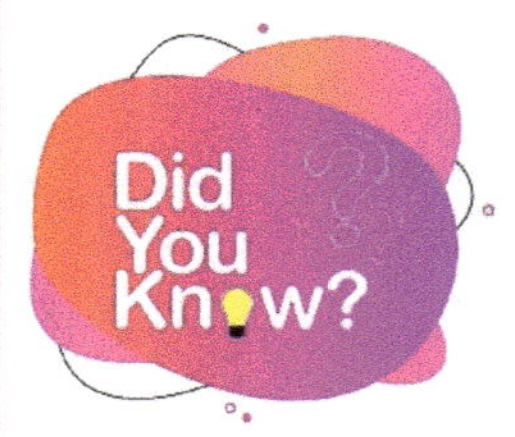

Some pregnant women feel like eating clay or chalk!

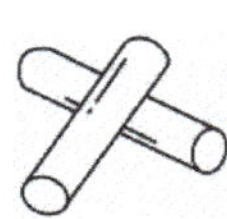

You read that right! This is referred to as pica. Pica is the practice of craving substances with little or no nutritional value. Dirt, clay, and laundry starch are the most common substances craved during pregnancy. Soap, plaster, paints, buttons, clay, hair, cigarette, pencil chewing, chalk, paper, gum, and coal – to name a few – could also be part of the list. Some women feel compelled to consume raw food items like flour, potatoes, rice, salt, peas, corn starch, etc.[15,16]

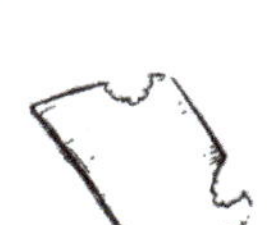

Why is it that pregnant women develop such cravings? While there is no exact cause we can put our finger on, it has been speculated to be linked to iron deficiency. Pica cravings are thought of as the body's attempt to obtain vitamins or minerals missing in the diet.[15]

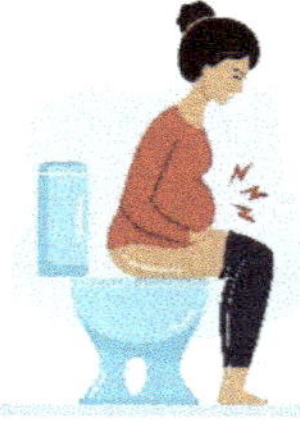

Sadly, the downside of pica is that it may harm the mom-to-be and/or the growing baby—consumption of substances containing lead, like paints and varnishes, results in lead poisoning and brain damage. Certain substances can harm the digestive system, causing constipation, ulceration, obstruction, nausea, abdominal distention, and loss of appetite. Pica can also pave the way for infections and parasitic infestations due to soil intake. It can also cause dental abnormalities, including severe tooth abrasion, abfraction, and surface tooth loss. Pica for paper (tissue boxes and cigarette packages) has also been reported to cause mercury poisoning.[15–17]

If it is this harmful, let's remedy this, shall we? [15,18,19]

- ✓ First and foremost, inform your healthcare provider. Testing and correcting nutrient deficiencies will be the first step in treating pica.
- ✓ On your part, you could try substitutes for the cravings, such as chewing sugarless gum, and get help from friends and family to avoid nonfood items.
- ✓ Sometimes, pica cravings may be related to an underlying mental illness. If pica does not stop even after nutritional interventions, worry not; maybe all you need is a big, warm hug to overcome the emotional roller coaster that accompanies pregnancy.
- ✓ And last but not least, there are also several behavioral interventions that you could consider.

Shape It Up

While many pregnant women have apprehensions about moving and grooving during their pregnancy, regular physical activity in all phases of life, including pregnancy, has health benefits. Pregnancy is an ideal time to adopt and/or maintain a healthy lifestyle.[20]

Look at all the brownie points you can earn by exercising during pregnancy.[20–22]

Improves mood & increases energy level
Promotes better sleep pattern
Reduces backaches , constipation, bloating, & swelling
YOGA
for
PREGNANT
Helps stay fit during pregnancy.
Easier to get back in shape after the baby is born.
Decrease the risk of gestational diabetes, preeclampsia, and caesarean delivery
Improves posture and promotes muscle tone, strength, & endurance
Promotes healthy weight gain during pregnancy
May improve the ability to cope with labour.

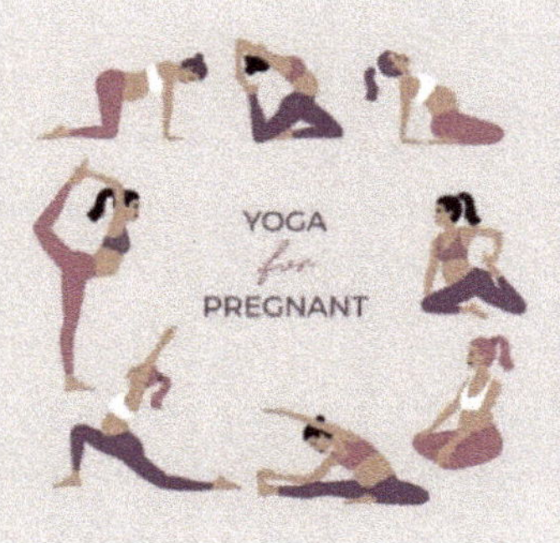

Is continuing or starting regular physical activity during a healthy, normal pregnancy safe? Contrary to what is feared, physical activity does not increase the risk of miscarriage, low birth weight, or early delivery. However, pregnant women with certain conditions or complications (premature labor, incompetent cervix/cerclage, multiple gestations at risk of premature birth, severe anaemia, etc.) may have to desist from exercising. Therefore, exercise must be started/continued during pregnancy only after your healthcare provider gives you a thumbs up.[22,23]

At least 150 minutes of moderate-intensity aerobic activity every week is recommended. Remember to be well-hydrated and avoid lying flat on the back for long periods. Here is an overview of safe and unsafe physical activities during pregnancy.[22,23]

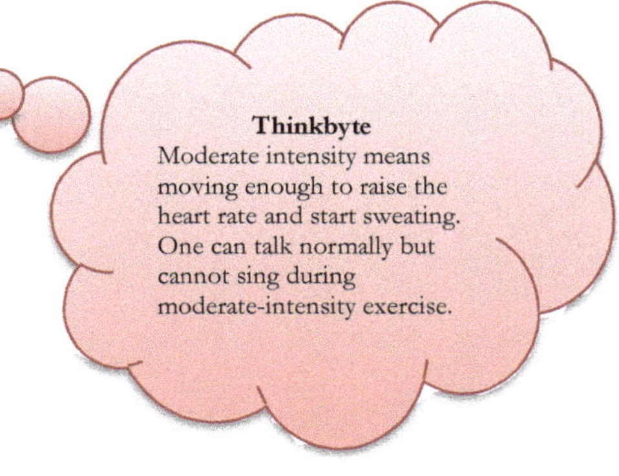

Safe physical activities[+]	Unsafe physical activities
Walking, swimming, stationary cycling, modified yoga*, running or jogging*, racquet sports[#], strength training*.	Ice hockey, boxing, soccer, basketball, suba diving, sky diving, hot yoga/pilates, activities with high risk of falling (skiing, surfing, horseback riding.

+In women with uncomplicated pregnancies in consultation with an obstetric care provider.
*Yoga positions that cause decreased venous return and hypotension must be avoided. Running, jogging, racquet sports, and strength training safe for those who participated regularly before pregnancy. Racquet sports involving changing balance and rapid movement to be avoided.

If you even have the slightest clue of the following symptoms, step away from your exercise mat and contact your healthcare provider:[22,23]

- ✗ Vaginal bleeding
- ✗ Dizziness

- ✗ Shortness of breath before starting exercise
- ✗ Chest pain
- ✗ Headache
- ✗ Muscle weakness
- ✗ Calf pain or swelling
- ✗ Regular, painful contractions of the uterus
- ✗ Fluid gushing or leaking from the vagina

Key Takeaways

- Optimal weight gain during pregnancy is essential to support and nurture both the mother and the growing foetus.
- Foetal growth and pregnancy demand additional nutrients.
- Healthcare providers along with qualified dieticians/nutritionists can draw up a tailored diet plan to ensure optimal nutrition during pregnancy.
- At least 150 minutes of moderate-intensity aerobic activity every week is recommended for a healthy, normal pregnancy.

Desirable Weight Gain During Pregnancy

Are you not a fan of formulas and calculations? No worries, you can quickly check if your weight gain is appropriate. You can even track it throughout your pregnancy! Just plot the weight you've gained against the week of pregnancy you're at.

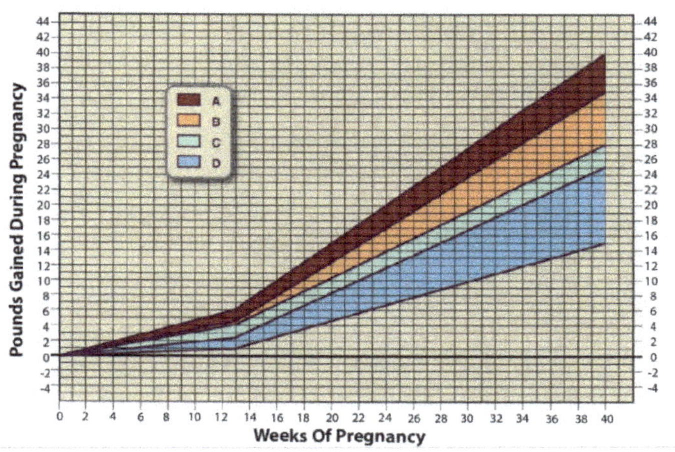

Adapted from: Kathleen Mahan, Sylvia Escott-Stump. Nutrition and Diagnosis-related Care. Edition 8. Wolters Kluwer Escott-Stump. Krause's Food, Nutrition, & Diet Therapy. Edition 12. W.B. Saunders

Here's how you get to know where you stand:

- Women of average weight before their pregnancy should aim for a weight gain in the B to C range (25–35 lb) during pregnancy.
- Underweight women should gain in the A to B range (28–40 lb).
- Overweight women should gain in the D range (15–25 lb).

References

1. Staci Nix. William's Basic Nutrition and Diet Therapy. 14 edn. Elviser: India, 2010.

2. Carol J. Lammi-Keefe. Handbook of Nutrition and Pregnancy. 2nd edn. Humana Press: New Jersey, 2018.
3. Institute of Medicine (US) and National Research Council (US) Committee to Reexamine IOM Pregnancy Weight Guidelines; Rasmussen KM, Yaktine AL, editors. Weight Gain During Pregnancy: Reexamining the Guidelines. Washington (DC): National Academies Press (US); 2009. Summary. Available from: https://www.ncbi.nlm.nih.gov/books/NBK32799/. It was accessed on 26 August 2019.
4. Luke B, Hediger ML, Nugent C, *et al.* Body mass index-specific weight gains associated with optimal birth weights in twin pregnancies. *J Reprod Med.* 2003;48:217–24.
5. Sylvia Escott-Stump. Nutrition and Diagnosis-related Care. 8th edn. Wolters Kluwer: Netherlands, 2015.
6. Kathleen Mahan, Sylvia Escott-Stump. Nutrition and Diagnosis-related Care. Edition 8. Wolters Kluwer Escott-Stump. Krause's Food, Nutrition, & Diet Therapy. Edition 12. W.B. Saunders.
7. ACOG. Nutrition During Pregnancy. Available at: https://www.acog.org/Patients/FAQs/Nutrition-During-Pregnancy. Accessed on 30 August 2019.
8. Kominiarek MA, Rajan P. Nutrition Recommendations in Pregnancy and Lactation. *Med Clin North Am.* 2016;100(6):1199–1215.
9. Paul M. Insel. Discovering Nutrition. 4th edn. Jones & Bartlett Publishers: Massachusetts, 2013.
10. Aparna P, Muthathal S, Nongkynrih B, *et al.* Vitamin D deficiency in India. *J Family Med Prim Care.* 2018;7(2):324–330.
11. NHS. How to get vitamin D from sunlight. Available at: https://www.nhs.uk/live-well/healthy-body/how-to-get-vitamin-d-from-sunlight/. Accessed on 30 August 2019.

12. Food Taboos During Pregnancy and Lactation Across the World. Available at: https://sightandlife.org/wp-content/uploads/2017/02/Food-Taboos-infographic.pdf. It was accessed on 26 August 2019.
13. BBC report. The myths about food and pregnancy. Available at: https://www.bbc.com/news/magazine-32033409. It was accessed on 26 August 2019.
14. National geography. Eat This, Not That: Taboos and Pregnancy. Available at: https://www.nationalgeographic.com/people-and-culture/food/the-plate/2015/03/19/eat-this-not-that-taboos-and-pregnancy/. Accessed on: 26 August 2019.
15. American Pregnancy Association. Pregnancy And Pica. Available at: https://americanpregnancy.org/pregnancy-health/unusual-cravings-pica/. Accessed on 26 August 2019.
16. Munir S. Qadir I M. Pathophysiology and management of pica. *Pharmacologyonline*. 2010;3:677–681.
17. Johnson BE. Pica. In: Walker HK, Hall WD, Hurst JW, editors. Clinical Methods: The History, Physical, and Laboratory Examinations. 3rd edition. Boston: Butterworths; 1990. Chapter 148. Available from: https://www.ncbi.nlm.nih.gov/books/NBK255/. It was accessed on 26 August 2019.
18. NEDA. PICA. Available at: https://www.nationaleatingdisorders.org/learn/by-eating-disorder/other/pica. Accessed on 26 August 2019.
19. Diet in pregnancy. Managing food cravings during pregnancy. Available at: https://www.dietinpregnancy.co.uk/pregnancy/pregnancy-cravings/. It was accessed on 26 August 2019.
20. American Pregnancy Association. Exercise during pregnancy. Available at: https://americanpregnancy.org/pregnancy-

health/exercise-during-pregnancy/. Accessed on 26 August 2019.

21. Berghella V, Saccone G. Exercise in pregnancy! *AJOG.* 2017;216(4):335–337.
22. ACOG. Exercise during pregnancy. Available at: https://www.acog.org/Patients/FAQs/Exercise-During-Pregnancy?IsMobileSet=false. Accessed on 26 August 2019.
23. Committee on Obstetric Practice. Physical Activity and Exercise During Pregnancy and the Postpartum Period. Available at: https://www.acog.org/Clinical-Guidance-and-Publications/Committee-Opinions/Committee-on-Obstetric-Practice/Physical-Activity-and-Exercise-During-Pregnancy-and-the-Postpartum-Period?IsMobileSet=false. Accessed on: 26 August 2019.

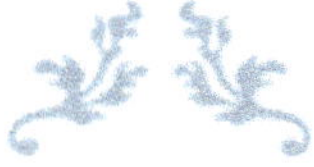

Getting to know that your baby has a defective spinal cord during pregnancy – or finding out that something is wrong with your baby – can be devastating. All your hopes and dreams for the little one go topsy-turvy. It's scary, saddening, and frustrating. This is the tragedy that Amy had witnessed her friend go through when she was 16 weeks into her third pregnancy. The whole story flashed before Amy's eyes as the doctor advised her about the importance of folic acid. She knew it wasn't to be taken lightly.

So what is the connection between folic acid and a baby's spinal cord development you ask? Let's find out.

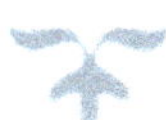

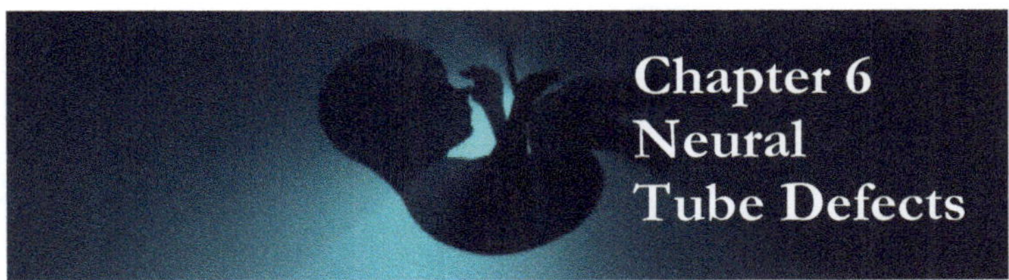

Chapter 6 Neural Tube Defects

First off, what are neural tube defects? While it may sound a bit complex, neural tube defects (NTDs) refer to the faulty brain and spinal cord development that is present at birth.[1]

A baby's neural tube (the starting material of the brain and spinal cord) starts as a tiny, flat ribbon and forms a tube by the end of

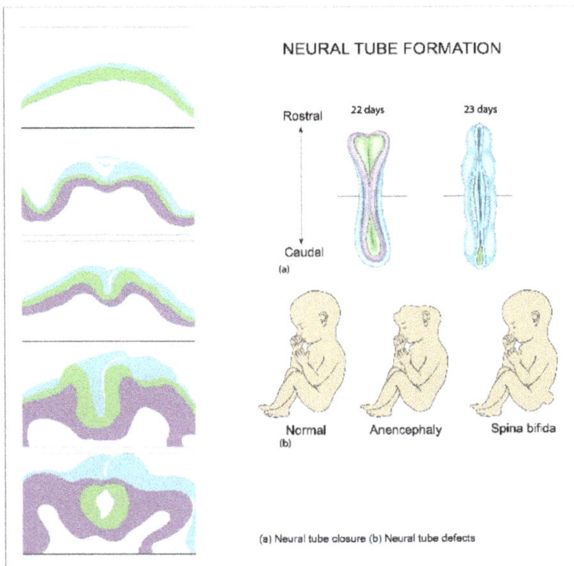

(a) Neural tube closure (b) Neural tube defects

the first month of pregnancy. In the event of incomplete closure of this tube, an NTD occurs. Unfortunately, NTDs not only cause serious problems for babies, but they are fatal as well. Spina bifida and anencephaly are the two most common NTDs.[1]

In spina bifida, the small bones of the spine do not close completely, and a part of the spinal cord protrudes through the spine. Children born with this condition may have paralyzed legs and bladder and bowel movement issues.[1]

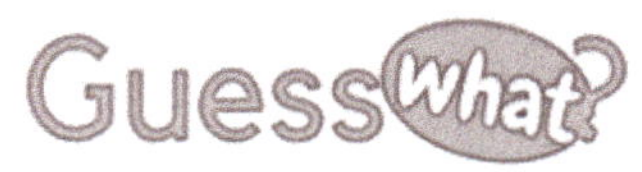

As recently as fifty years ago, the cause of NTDs was not known. British researchers found that mothers of children with spina bifida had low vitamin levels, more than 30 years ago. Eventually, two studies demonstrated that poor maternal folate levels were linked to NTDs.[5]

Anencephaly is caused due to the incomplete closure of the upper part of the neural tube that forms the brain. Consequently, babies with this condition lack central brain, skull, and scalp parts. Regrettably, they survive for just a few hours after birth.[1]

Prenatal tests or screening tests, viz. medical tests conducted during pregnancy (such as blood tests and ultrasound), help detect NTDs.[1,2]

Deterring the Debacle Through Folic Acid Supplementation

Remember that a woman's nutritional status before and during pregnancy has a crucial impact on foetal growth and development. Notably, poor nutritional status before conception and during early pregnancy (up to 12 weeks gestation) increases the risk of adverse pregnancy outcomes.[3]

Research shows that folic acid supplementation in the periconceptional period (before and during pregnancy), alone or in combination with other vitamins and minerals, helps prevent NTDs.[3] Most women miss out on folic acid supplementation until they are pregnant, which is too late for the effective prevention of NTDs.[4]

According to the World Health Organization, "All women, from the moment they begin trying to conceive until 12 weeks of gestation, should take a folic acid supplement (400 µg folic acid daily)." Moreover, women who have had a baby diagnosed with an NTD or have given birth to a baby with an NTD must: [3]

- Be offered high-dose supplementation (5 mg folic acid daily)
- Be advised to increase their food intake of folate

The Centers for Disease Control and Prevention (CDC) also recommends that folic acid supplementation of 400 µg/day for all women of reproductive age, in addition to the consumption of food with folate from a varied diet, to help prevent NTDs.[6]

Naturally occurring folic acid is called folate. Beans (like lentils, pinto beans, and black beans), leafy green vegetables (like spinach and romaine lettuce), asparagus, broccoli, peanuts, and citrus fruits (like oranges and grapefruit) are good sources of folate.[1]

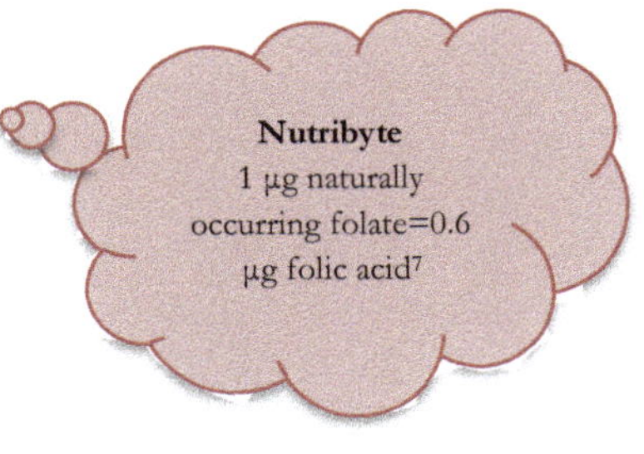

Bear in mind that obtaining the requisite folic acid solely from food is challenging. Hence, adding a daily vitamin supplement is advisable.[1]

The following illustration will give you an idea of how much folate is present in common foods:[7]

1 SMALL ORANGE 29 µg
1 MEDIUM BANANA 24 µg
1 LARGE EGG 22 µg
2 SLICES OF WHITE BREAD 64 µg
4 BOILED ASPARAGUS SPEARS 89 µg

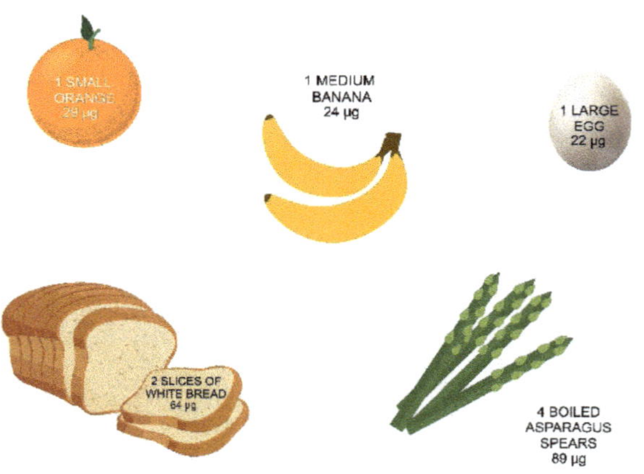

Listed below are a few more folate-rich foods, along with their folate content: [7]

Food item	Folate (µg/serving)
Beef liver, braised, 3 ounces	215
Spinach, boiled, ½ cup	131
Black-eyed peas (cowpeas), cooked, ½ cup	105

Brussels sprouts, frozen, boiled, ½ cup	78
Lettuce, romaine, shredded, 1 cup	64
Avocado, raw, sliced, ½ cup	59
Spinach, raw, 1 cup	58
Broccoli, chopped, frozen, cooked, ½ cup	52
Mustard greens, chopped, frozen, boiled, ½ cup	52
Green peas, frozen, boiled, ½ cup	47
Kidney beans, canned, ½ cup	46
Wheat germ, two tablespoons	40
Tomato juice, canned, ¾ cup	36
Crab, Dungeness, 3 ounces	36
Orange juice, ¾ cup	35
Turnip greens, frozen, boiled, ½ cup	32
Peanuts, dry roasted, 1 ounce	27
Papaya, raw, cubed, ½ cup	27
Yeast, baker's, ¼ teaspoon	23
Cantaloupe, raw, cubed, ½ cup	17
Vegetarian baked beans, canned, ½ cup	15
Fish, halibut, cooked, 3 ounces	12

Milk, 1% fat, 1 cup	12
Ground beef, 85% lean, cooked, 3 ounces	7
Chicken breast, roasted, 3 ounces	3

In some countries, foods such as breads, breakfast cereals, flour, cornmeal, pasta, rice, and other grain products are fortified or enriched with folic acid. These products can also increase folic acid intake.[1,7]

Tackling Neural Tube Defects: Beyond Folic Acid Supplementation

Low fruit and vegetable intake has been linked to an elevated risk of NTDs. Since fruits and vegetables are rich in folate, low intake of these foods may be associated with inadequate folate intake.[4]

Recent research has revealed that poor status of vitamin B_2, B_6, B_{12}, choline, betaine, or omega-3 fats is associated with an increased risk of NTDs. Thus, multivitamin B combined with choline, betaine, and *omega*-3 fat supplementation may have a better protective effect against NTDs than folic acid alone. However, further research is required to confirm this.[4]

Study findings indicate that tea consumption increases the risk of NTDs even in women whose folic acid intake exceeds 400 µg. It has been hypothesized that tea consumption might interfere with folate metabolism and cause NTDs. Similarly, coffee consumption has also been associated with a hike in NTD risk.

Thus, limiting the intake of caffeinated beverages may be beneficial for preventing NTDs.

Last but not least, alcohol consumption may result in low blood folate levels. Hence, it may be beneficial if alcohol intake is limited among women of childbearing age.[4]

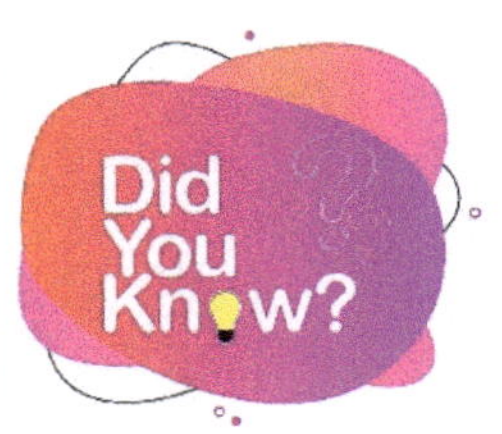

Obesity and diabetes can also increase the likelihood of NTDs... Yikes!

Researchers have unearthed that high body fat and a body mass index (BMI) of 30 or higher (in other words, being obese) increase the risk of conceiving a baby with an NTD. Aiming for a healthy weight before pregnancy is the way forward.[1]

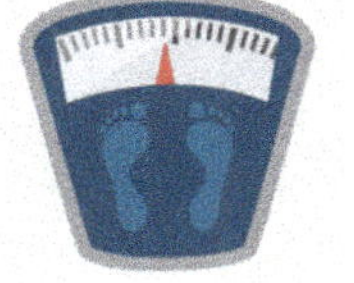

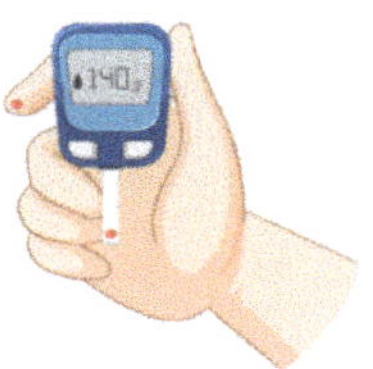

Uncontrolled diabetes (a condition involving high blood glucose levels) also increases the risk of NTDs in a baby. If you have diabetes, keep your blood glucose levels in check by adhering to an appropriate diet and exercise regimen.[1]

Key Takeaways

- Incomplete closure of the neural tube in a developing baby leads to an NTD. Spina bifida and anencephaly are the two most common NTDs.
- Folic acid supplementation in the periconceptional period (before and during pregnancy), either alone or in combination with other vitamins and minerals, helps prevent neural tube defects.
- Four hundred μg/day of folic acid supplementation for all women of reproductive age, in addition to consuming food with folate from a varied diet, is recommended to help prevent NTDs.
- Most women miss out on folic acid supplementation until they are pregnant, which is too late for the effective prevention of NTDs.
- Women of childbearing age must avoid tea, coffee, and alcohol; doing so may be beneficial in preventing NTDs.
- Aiming for a healthy weight and keeping blood glucose levels under control prior to pregnancy can also help reduce the risk of NTDs.

Spot it!

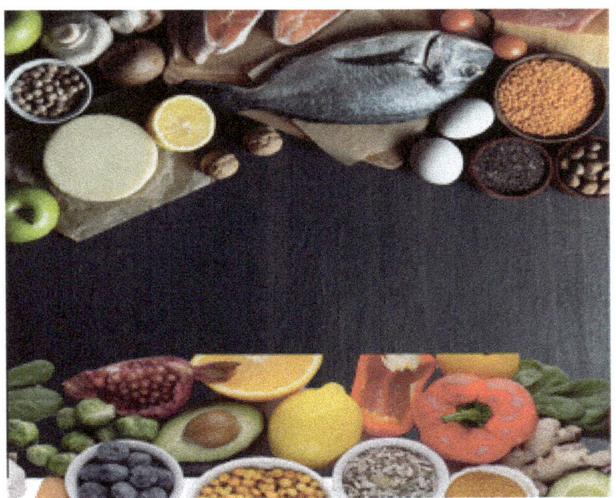

Check and see if you can spot folate-rich foods.

Answers: Beef, spinach, egg, avocado, beans and lentils, broccoli

References

1. March of Dimes. Neural Tube Defects. Available at: https://www.marchofdimes.org/complications/neural-tube-defects.aspx. It was accessed on 04 September 2019.
2. National Institute of Child Health and Human Development. Neural Tube Defects. Available at: https://www.nichd.nih.gov/health/topics/ntds/conditioninfo/diagnosed. It was accessed on 04 September 2019.
3. WHO. Periconceptional folic acid supplementation to prevent neural tube defects. Available at:

https://www.who.int/elena/titles/folate_periconceptional/en/. It was accessed on 04 September 2019.

4. Li K, Wahlqvist ML, Li D. Nutrition, one-carbon metabolism, and neural tube defects: A review. *Nutrients*. 2016;8(11):741.
5. Harvard T.H. Chan School of Public Health. Folate (Folic Acid). Available at: https://www.hsph.harvard.edu/nutritionsource/folic-acid/. It was accessed on 04 September 2019.
6. CDC. Folic acid. Available at: https://www.cdc.gov/ncbddd/folicacid/recommendations.html. Accessed on: 04 September 2019.
7. NHS. Folate. Fact Sheet for Health Professionals. Available at: https://ods.od.nih.gov/factsheets/Folate-HealthProfessional/. Accessed on: 04 September 2019.

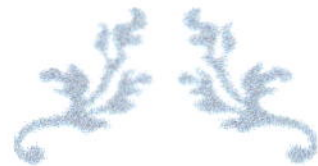

Sara was into her twentieth week of pregnancy and had come for her first ultrasound scan. She was very upbeat about her pregnancy as the scan showed that she was pregnant with twins.

As she was a career-oriented woman, Sara had long delayed her plans of expanding her family. She was 41 years old and had been apprehensive about getting pregnant. The news of the twins excited her and her husband. Sara was on cloud nine.

Sara made a visit to her gynaecologist with the scan report. Her happiness did not last long, as her doctor told her that she might be having hypertension that is mostly associated with pregnancy. Prior to conception, she was fairly healthy. It was only then that she realised that her sister too had gestational hypertension and had delivered a premature baby. She found it hard to accept the situation. Her doctor reassured her and suggested her to follow up after 15 days with her urine report.

Luckily, she did not have proteinuria (an excessive amount of protein in the urine). Her doctor advised her to reduce the intake of salt and follow a healthy diet. Despite her doctor's assurance, she began to worry about her pregnancy. Besides a counsellor, her doctor referred her to a nutritionist. As she did not want anything to cause harm to her babies, Sara was ready to follow the recommendations made by her doctor and nutritionist diligently....

Well, what kind of a diet is suitable for patients with or at risk of pregnancy-induced hypertension?

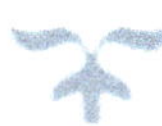

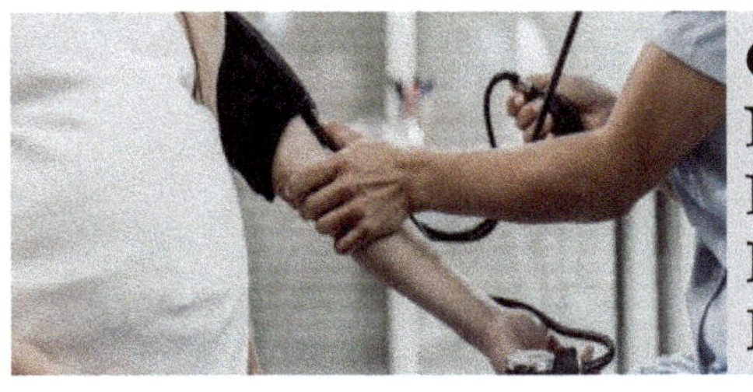

Chapter 7 Nutrition and Pregnancy-Induced Hypertension

Pregnancy-induced hypertension (PIH), also known as gestational hypertension, is a condition wherein the blood pressure rises to 140/90 mmHg or more during pregnancy. This can either be due to pre-existing hypertension or hypertension that develops after the twentieth week of gestation. Interestingly, pre-existing hypertension can sometimes coexist with gestational hypertension and proteinuria (presence of protein in urine).[1] When proteinuria hypertension team up, the condition is then called preeclampsia.[2]

Pregnancy-induced hypertension is a grave concern for the mother, the foetus, and the newborn baby. Like a ghost lurking in the shadows, PIH may exist, and women may not be aware of its presence at all, making PIH particularly harmful in its early stages. Moreover, it can adversely impact pregnancy outcomes.[3] Pregnancy-induced hypertension is a multiorgan disease and is seen to affect the heart and its vessels (cardiovascular), the kidneys, the brain and spinal cord, and the liver.[4]

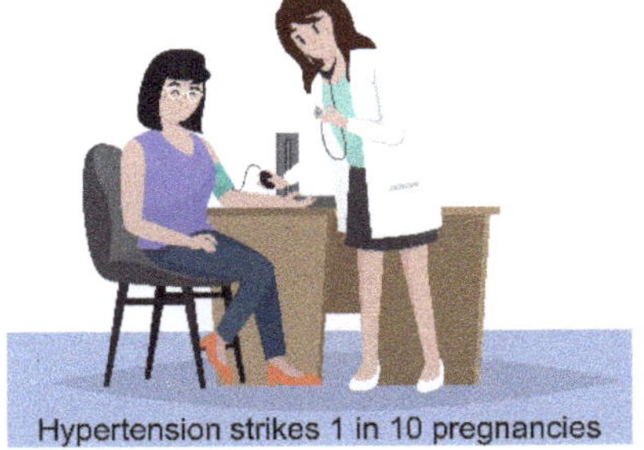

Hypertension strikes 1 in 10 pregnancies

Poor Diet and PIH/Preeclampsia: The Connexion

While several medical conditions, such as pre-existing hypertension and cardiovascular disease, increase the risk for a pregnant woman to develop PIH, certain nutritional factors can also be contributing factors.[2,5] More specifically, obesity and excessive weight gain during pregnancy could cause preeclampsia.[6] Researchers have unearthed that the risk of PIH is linked to a diet that primarily comprises fast food, characterized by the increased consumption of potatoes, mixed meat, margarine, and white bread.[5]

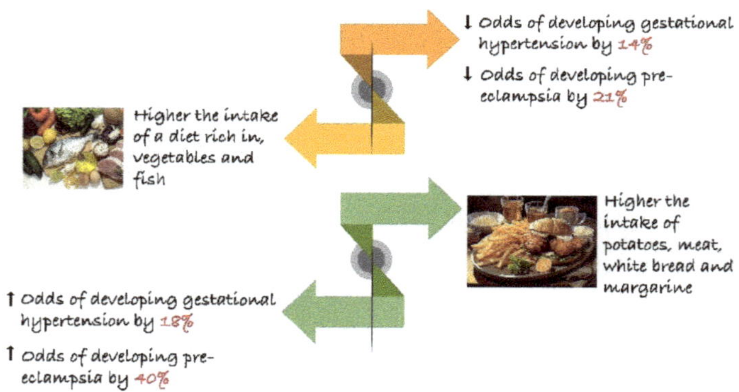

It is believed that low protein intake is associated with an increased risk of developing preeclampsia as well. A dietary pattern that includes a reduced intake of good fats, especially omega-3 and omega-6 fatty acids, and a high intake of long-chain polyunsaturated fatty acids has been observed among women with gestational hypertension.[7]

Evidence from studies suggests that the lack of certain micronutrients is linked to the development of PIH. Mothers on an energy-rich diet, low in magnesium and calcium, are at risk of developing PIH or preeclampsia.[8] Zinc concentrations are lower among women with preeclampsia, suggesting an association between preeclampsia and zinc level.[7] Likewise, low vitamin D levels increase the risk of preeclampsia.[9]

Optimal Diet: Need of the Hour in Preeclampsia/PIH

While nothing can be done regarding certain risk factors such as genetics, diet, and lifestyle, they are risk factors that lie in our own hands. Look at a few small diet and lifestyle changes that can help prevent PIH.

Ways to keep pregnancy induced hypertension at bay!
Keeping the feet elevates several times during the day
Consuming at least 8 glasses of water a day
Exercising regularly
Avoiding alcohol and beverages containing caffeine
Limiting intake of salt
Healthy measures
Increasing protein in diet and decreasing fries foods and junk food you eat
Ensuring good amount of rest

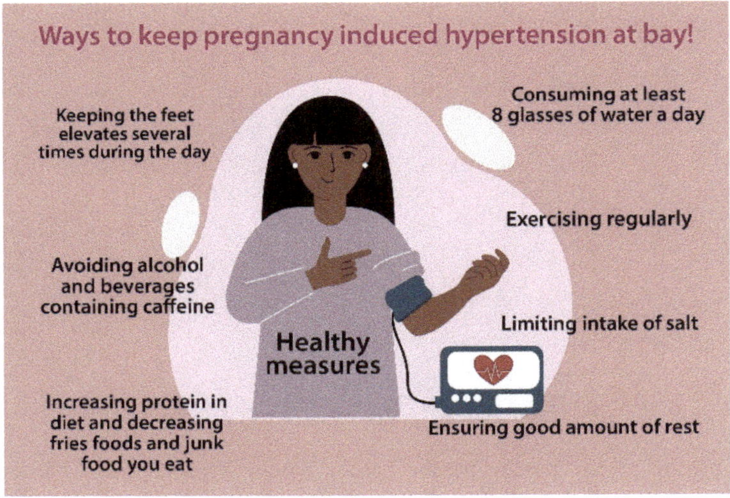

A balanced diet with optimal calories in high-quality protein (a protein well absorbed and utilized by the body, like egg protein), calcium, potassium, vitamin A, iron, and folic acid-rich foods is recommended for women with PIH.[10] The diet should contain an optimum amount of sodium. Recent research shows that the body needs salt during pregnancy to maintain a proper fluid balance.[6,11] Organic produce, viz., food grown without pesticides, fertilizers, or genetically modified organisms, reduces the risk of developing preeclampsia.[12] Presumably, the protective role of organic food is due to low exposure to dietary pesticides, higher intake of secondary plant metabolites, and perhaps a different microflora (tiny organisms) on organic vegetables with a potentially beneficial effect.[12]

Nutritional Advice for Pregnant Women From the Royal College Of Obstetricians And Gynaecologists

Women must consider these few steps towards healthy eating during pregnancy:[13]

- Eat at least five portions of different fruits and vegetables daily instead of foods high in fat and calories. Never include potatoes in the count of the five–day target.
- Meals should contain starchy foods, such as potatoes, bread, rice, and pasta, but it is wise to choose whole grains as far as possible.
- A low-fat diet should be considered. Never think of increasing the number of calories you eat.
- Treat yourself to very little fried food, but avoid drinks high in added sugars and foods such as sweets and cakes. Instead, turn your platter into fibre-rich foods, such as oats, beans, lentils, grains, seeds, wholegrain bread, brown rice, and wholemeal pasta.

- Include protein in your diet every day; choose lean meat and try to eat two portions of fish a week. If you are a vegetarian, lentils, beans, and tofu are the protein sources that you would need.

- Do not "eat for two". Watch the portion size of your meals and snacks, and note how often you eat.

- Do not skip breakfast.

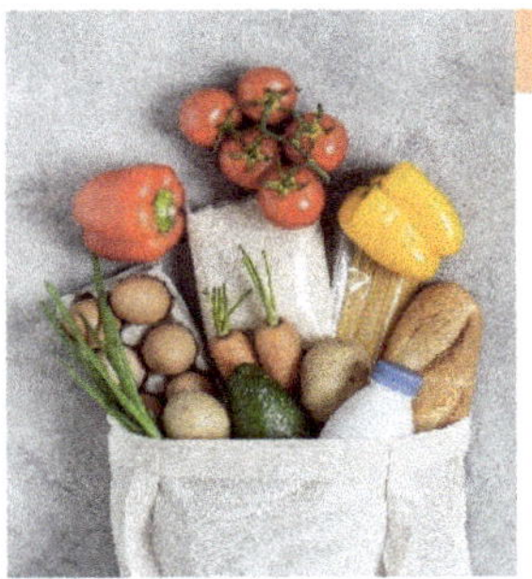

Danish National Birth Cohort

Higher the intake of a diet rich in vegetables and fish Lower is the risk for hypertension during pregnancy.

Nutritional Supplementation for Preeclampsia/PIH

Oxidative stress in the development of preeclampsia. As a result, antioxidant vitamin supplements, in combination with L-arginine supplements during pregnancy, dramatically reduce the incidence of preeclampsia, especially among those who are at risk of developing preeclampsia.[6] Lycopene, another antioxidant, has also been found to prevent the development of preeclampsia.[5] Other potent antioxidants that could be beneficial

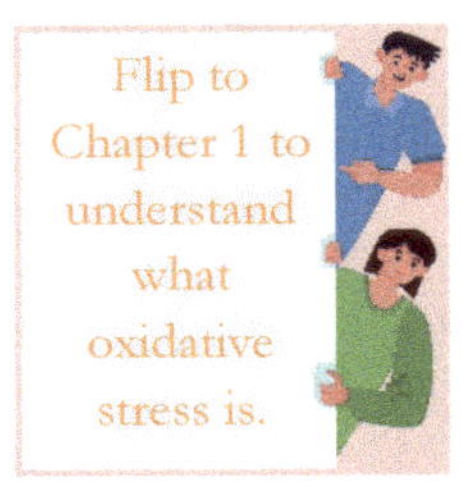

are carotenoids, such as α-carotene, β-carotene, and canthaxanthin.[7]

The People's Health League study confirmed the benefits of micronutrient supplementation and halibut liver oil from the twentieth week of pregnancy for reducing the risk of developing preeclampsia.[7,14] Omega-3 fatty acids could also be a feasible option! [15]

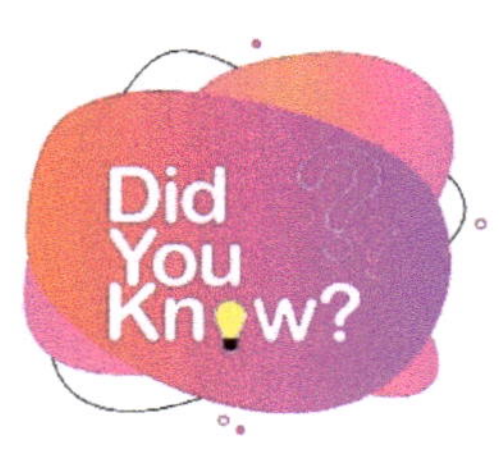

Fish is not just rich in protein and omega-3 but also mercury!

Fish is famous for its omega-3 content; however, not all fish are good for pregnancy. The beneficial effects of omega-3 fats can be overthrown by the presence of mercury and other harmful toxins (such as polychlorinated biphenyls [PCBs]).[16,17]

Mercury in fish can increase the risk of cardiovascular diseases and hinder neurological development. Hence, potentially conflicting reports question the risks and benefits of fish consumption in adults.[18]

Considering the pros and cons of fish as a dietary source of omega-3 fats, the US Food and Drug Administration and Environmental Protection Agency recommends limiting fish consumption to two servings (approximately 340 g or 12 oz of seafood) per week.[16]

Choose species that are high in omega-3 fatty acids and low in mercury. These include salmon, trout, and shrimp. Avoid species with high mercury levels and omega-3 fatty acids, including tuna, shark, halibut, swordfish, and sea bass.[18]

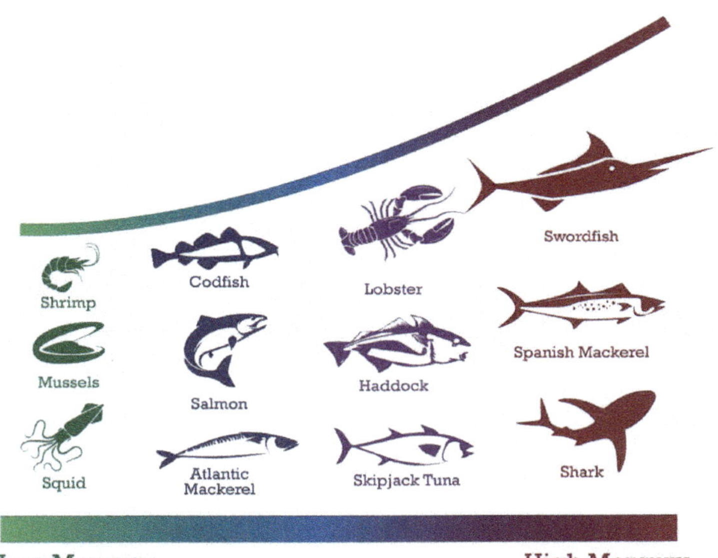

Adapted from Nature's Academy. The Issue with Fish Tissue. Available at: https://www.naturesacademy.org/environmental-awareness/the-issue-with-fish-tissue/. It was accessed on 06 September 2019.

Considering that calcium metabolism is likely to be affected by PIH, calcium supplementation could reduce the chances of developing gestational hypertension.[19] Pregnant women having a low level of calcium benefit from calcium supplementation in terms of lowering the incidence of preeclampsia or PIH.[7] Significant reductions in diastolic blood pressure have also been achieved following calcium supplementation in those with gestational hypertension.[19]

Key Takeaways

- Pregnancy-induced hypertension is a grave concern. It affects the heart and it vessels (cardiovascular), the kidneys, the brain and spinal cord, and the liver
- Pregnancy-induced hypertension is likely to have a long-term adverse impact on the mother and the newborn child.
- Pregnancy-induced hypertension is linked to a diet that mainly comprises fast food, characterised by the increased consumption of potatoes, mixed meat, margarine, and white bread.
- Antioxidant and micronutrient supplementation demonstrate potential benefits for PIH.

Crossword Puzzle – Diet and Pregnancy-Induced Hypertension

Take out your pens and get solving!

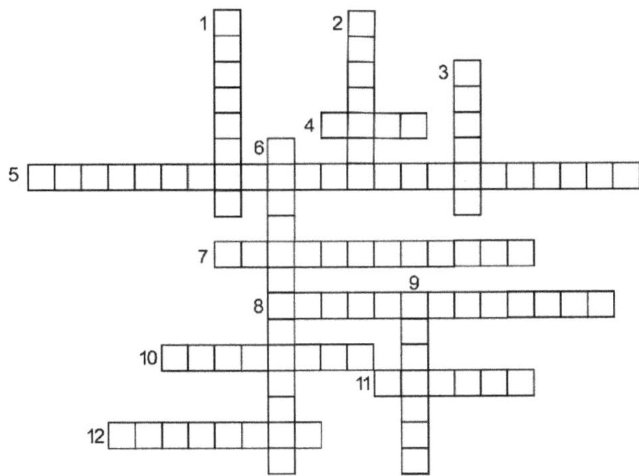

Down:

1. A diet comprised of potatoes, mixed meat, margarine and white bread (4,4)
2. Not all fishes are deemed good for pregnancy because of high levels of ____________ (7)

Across:

4. A fish high in mercury and omega-3 fatty acids (4)

6. A blood pressure of 140/50 mmHg or more during pregnancy (12)

7. Hypertension plus protein in urine (proteinuria) in pregnancy (12)

8. ________ and ________ helpful in improving anemia

3. A tuber not be considered in court of five-a-day target of vegetables and fruits (6) 5. Women with preeclampsia are more likely to be deficient in ________ and ________ minerals found in shell fish (9.4) 9. Foods with low exposure to pesticides (7)	also reduces the risk of preeclampsia (4,5,4) 10. Vitamin deficiency that increases the risk of pre-eclampsia (7,1) 11. A fish high in omega-3 fatty acids and low in mercury (6) 12. Antioxidant found in tomator that could take of preeclampsia (8)

Answers to crosswords

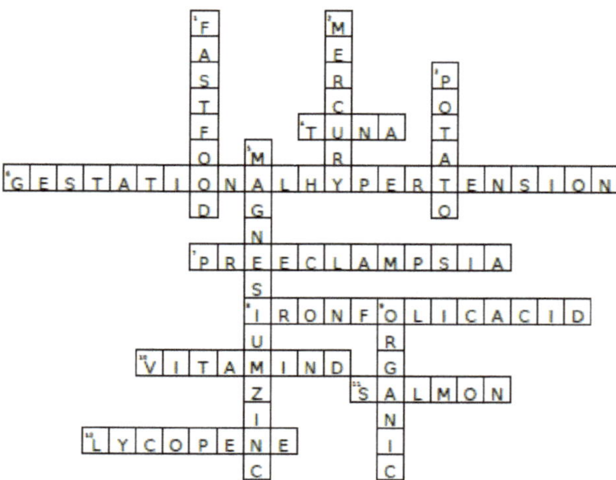

References

1. Kintiraki E, Papakatsika S, Kotronis G. Pregnancy-Induced hypertension. *Hormones (Athens).* 2015;14(2):211–223.
2. American Pregnancy Association. Gestational Hypertension: Pregnancy-Induced Hypertension (PIH). Available at: https://americanpregnancy.org/pregnancy-complications/pregnancy-induced-hypertension/. Accessed on 20 August 2019.
3. Maputle S, Khoza L, Lebese R. Knowledge towards pregnancy-induced hypertension among pregnant women in Vhembe District, Limpopo Province. *J Hum Ecol.* 2015;51(1,2):47–54.
4. Chuang CH, Velott DL, Weisman CS. Exploring knowledge and attitudes related to pregnancy and preconception health in women with chronic medical conditions. *Matern Child Health J.* 2010;14(5):713–719.
5. Iklem E, Halldorsson TI, Birgisdottir BE, *et al.* Dietary patterns and the risk of pregnancy-associated hypertension in the Danish National Birth Cohort: A prospective longitudinal study. BJOG. 2019;126:663–673.
6. Rasouli M, Pourheidari M, Hamzeh Gardesh Z. Effect of self-care before and during pregnancy to prevention and control preeclampsia in high-risk women. *Int J Prev Med.* 2019;10:21.
7. Roberts JM, Balk JL, Bodnar LM, *et al.* Nutrient involvement in preeclampsia. *J Nutrit.* 2003;133(5): 1684S–1692S.
8. Schoenake DAJM, Soedamah-Muthu SS, Mishra GD. The association between dietary factors and gestational

hypertension and pre-eclampsia: A systematic review and meta-analysis of observational studies. *BMC Med.* 2014;12:157.

9. Tabesh M, Salehi-Abargouei A, Tabesh M, *et al.* Maternal vitamin D status and risk of pre-eclampsia: A systematic review and meta-analysis. *J Clin Endocrinol Metab.* 2013;98(8):3165–3173.
10. Agrawal S, Fledderjohann J, Vellakkal S, *et al.* Adequately diversified dietary intake and iron and folic acid supplementation during pregnancy are associated with reduced occurrence of symptoms suggestive of pre-eclampsia or eclampsia in Indian Women. *PLoS ONE.* 2015;10(3):e0119120
11. Dietary Guidelines for pregnancy-induced hypertension Available at: https://www.fernandezhospital.com/Uploads/Document/189/dietary_guidelines_for_pregnancy_induced_hypertension.pdf Accessed on 20 August 2019
12. Torjusen H, Brantsæter AL, Haugen M, *et al.* Reduced risk of pre-eclampsia with organic vegetable consumption: Results from the prospective Norwegian Mother and Child Cohort Study. *BMJ Open.* 2014;4:e006143. doi:10.1136/bmjopen-2014- 006143
13. RCOG statement: Advice on nutrition in pregnancy Available at: https://www.rcog.org.uk/en/news/rcog-statement-advice-on-nutrition-in-pregnancy/ Accessed on 1 September 2019
14. Olsen SF, Secher NJ. A possible preventive effect of low-dose fish oil on early delivery and pre-eclampsia: indications from a 50-year-old controlled trial. *Br J Nutr.* 1990;64(3):599–609.

15. Oken E, Ning Y, Rifas-Shiman SL, *et al.* Diet during pregnancy and risk of preeclampsia or gestational hypertension. *Ann Epidemiol.* 2007;17(9):663–668.
16. Coletta JM, Bell SJ, Roman AS. Omega-3 fatty acids and pregnancy. *Rev Obstet Gynecol.* 2010;3(4):163–171.
17. Smith KL, Guentzel JL. Mercury concentrations and omega-3 fatty acids in fish and shrimp: Preferential consumption for maximum health benefits. Mar *Pollut Bull.* 2010;60(9):1615–1618.
18. Park K, Mozaffarian D. Omega-3 fatty acids, mercury, and selenium in fish and the risk of cardiovascular diseases. *Curr Atheroscler Rep.* 2010;12(6):414–422.
19. Ritchie LD, King JC, Dietary calcium and pregnancy-induced hypertension: is there a relation? *Am J Clinic Nutrit.* 2000;71(5):1371S–1374S.

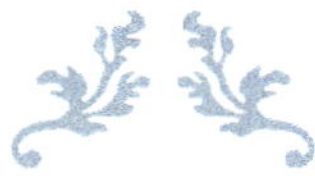

Anna was regular with her follow-ups and health check-ups. After her latest check-up, which included a one-hour glucose test, her doctor called her again for an additional test – her blood glucose levels appeared to be high. After a gruelling three-hour test, the results were out. Anna was benumbed to hear that she had gestational diabetes mellitus, a condition wherein blood glucose level is higher than normal.

To her relief, Anna learned from her doctor that gestational diabetes is a common condition. Lifestyle modifications and medications (if required) could help her ensure a healthy pregnancy and baby.

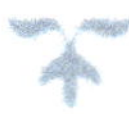

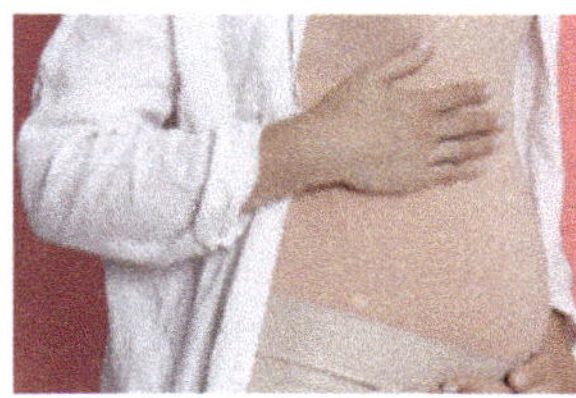

Chapter 8
Dealing With Gestational Diabetes Mellitus During Pregnancy

I was wondering what gestational diabetes mellitus (GDM) is. As the name suggests, gestational diabetes is a condition in which a woman who has not previously been diagnosed with diabetes exhibits high blood glucose levels during pregnancy.[1]

> **GDM affects almost 3%–5% of all pregnancies.[2]**

As seen in the image, insulin is the hormone your body cells require to utilize sugar from your blood.[2]

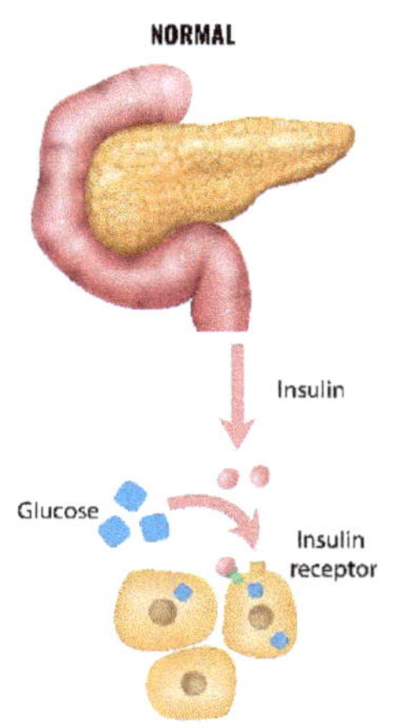

Lack of insulin prevents the use of sugar from the blood and results in high blood sugar levels.

TYPE 1 DIABETES
Insulin
Glucose

As pregnancy progresses, especially in the second and third trimesters, a surge of hormones, such as progesterone, cortisol, and placental growth hormone, causes insulin resistance. Moreover, the growing demands of the foetus increase the woman's insulin requirement. In a normal pregnancy, pancreatic cells responsible for insulin production (β cells) undergo proliferation (hyperplasia) to overcome insulin resistance. The inability to combat insulin resistance despite β-cell hyperplasia results in GDM. As body cells cannot utilise glucose without insulin, its levels in the blood increase.[1,2]

Are All Pregnant Women at Risk for GDM?

Any woman can develop gestational diabetes during pregnancy. However, a few factors increase your risk for GDM. According to research, the prevalence of GDM increases in tandem with an increase in the prevalence of obesity in women of childbearing age.[3] Other risk factors for GDM are as mentioned below.[1,4]

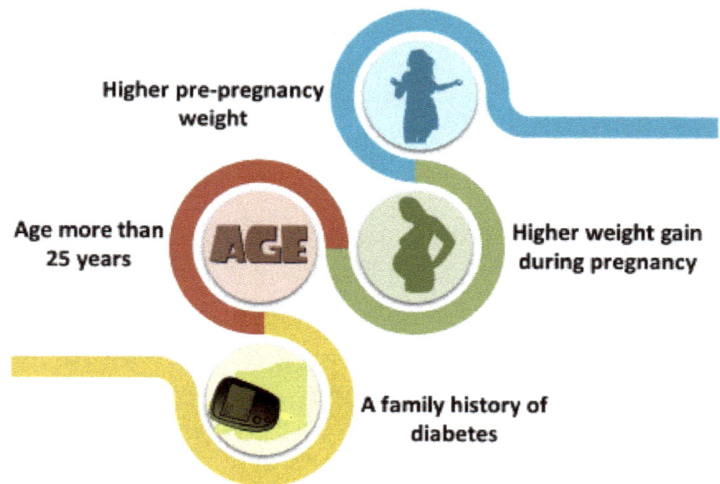

Most women with GDM will have a healthy pregnancy. However, in some cases, GDM can pose a risk to both the mother and child. A few complications associated with GDM are as follows:[5]

- Growth of the baby is more than usual
- Premature delivery
- Obstructed labour (dystocia)
- Baby developing jaundice after birth
- Too much amniotic fluid (the fluid surrounding the baby)
- An increased risk of type 2 diabetes in the future

According to the World Health Organization, a woman is diagnosed with GDM if she has any of the following: [6]

- Fasting blood glucose levels of 92–125 mg/dL
- 1-hour blood glucose levels after a 75-g oral glucose load of ≥180 mg/dL
- 2-hour blood glucose levels after a 75-g oral glucose load of 153–199 mg/dL

Science Behind GDM Management

If you have GDM, managing your blood glucose levels will help prevent the development of associated complications. Here are a few things you can do to manage your GDM effectively:

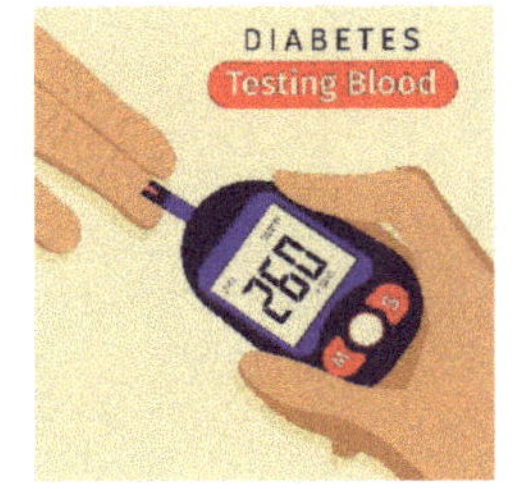

Finger prickin' good: Your doctor might ask you to monitor your blood glucose levels four to five times a day to ensure they remain within the healthy range. You might consider it tiresome and mundane, but it'll benefit you long term.[7]

To test your blood sugar level, draw a drop of blood using a lancet (a small needle), then place it on a test strip inserted into the blood glucose meter.[7]

Best foot forward: Make exercise your friend, as it will help you manage this ordeal. Exercise stimulates your body to move glucose into the cells, which are utilized for energy, lowering blood glucose levels. Exercise also increases your cells' response to insulin, improving insulin sensitivity. Relief from certain discomforts of pregnancy, such as trouble sleeping and back pain, is an added benefit of exercise.[7]

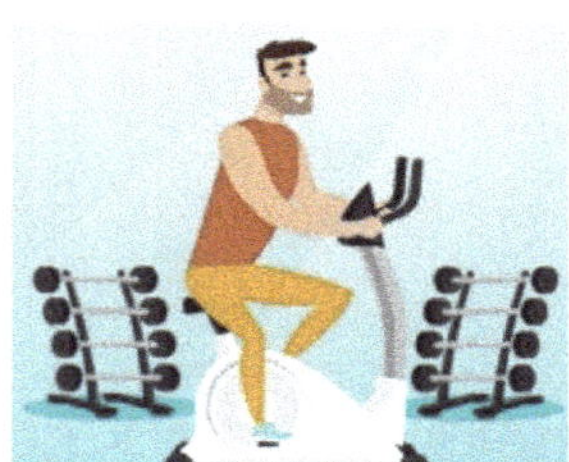

With your doctor's approval, aim for moderately vigorous exercise almost daily.[7]

Eat well… to be well!: Eating the correct food item in the right proportions is the key to keeping excessive weight gain at bay and controlling your blood glucose levels.[7]

A healthy diet focuses on items high in fibre and nutrition and low in calories and fats. Your doctor might recommend consulting a dietitian, who will provide you with a tailored meal plan.[7]

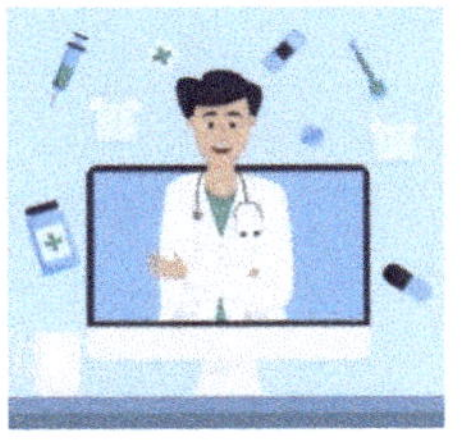

Do I need insulin?: If your doctor feels that diet and exercise alone aren't sufficient for you, they will advise insulin injections to manage your blood glucose levels.[7]

Nutrition Side to Managing GDM

A wholesome diet can help you maintain sound health and prevent complications for you and your baby. Three small-to-moderate-sized meals and two to four snacks per day are typically recommended for a woman with GDM. Meal plan adjustment is usually based on blood glucose levels, weight gain, appetite, and exercise schedule.[8]

In the case of insulin therapy, the primary meal plan goal is to maintain carbohydrate uniformity at snacks and meals to aid insulin adjustment.

With calories, don't go large; take charge!: The first step in any meal plan is deciding the calories required. (Read the box on the right to know more about calories.) Your dietitian will help you with this.[8]

Go light on carbs: Carbohydrates constitute the primary food group affecting blood glucose levels, and thus, their intake must be planned. The total amount of carbohydrates, type of carbohydrates, and distribution of carbohydrates throughout meals and snacks are considered. Usually, carbohydrate intake is limited to 40 percent of the total calorie intake.[8]

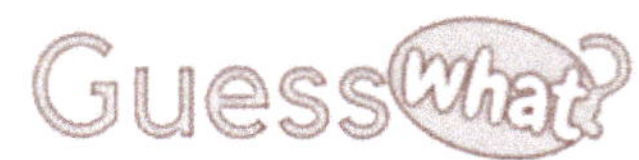

Everyone knows that including the right amount of calories is essential in any meal plan. But do you know how this is calculated for a woman with GDM? Well, it depends on the weight![8]

- For women with an ideal body weight, the caloric requirement is 30 kcal/kg/day.
- For those who are overweight, the caloric requirement is 25 kcal/kg/day.
- For women who are severely obese, the caloric requirement is 12 to 14 kcal/kg/day.
- For those who are underweight, the caloric requirement is 35 to 40 kcal/kg/day.

Pssssttt.......

As water contains no calories or carbohydrates, it is the best drink for anyone with GDM. It also aids in combating high blood glucose levels by triggering the kidneys to excrete sugar through urine![9]

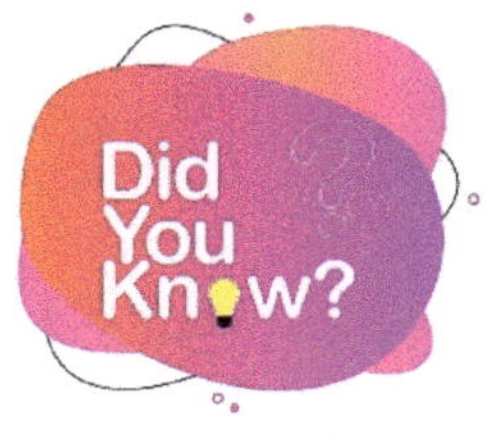

Glycaemic Index and Glycaemic Load Can Help Manage Your Sugar Levels! [10,11]

The glycaemic index (GI) ranks food items according to the rate at which they are broken down by the body to form glucose. So, high-GI foods are quickly broken down into glucose, whereas low-GI foods are broken down slowly.

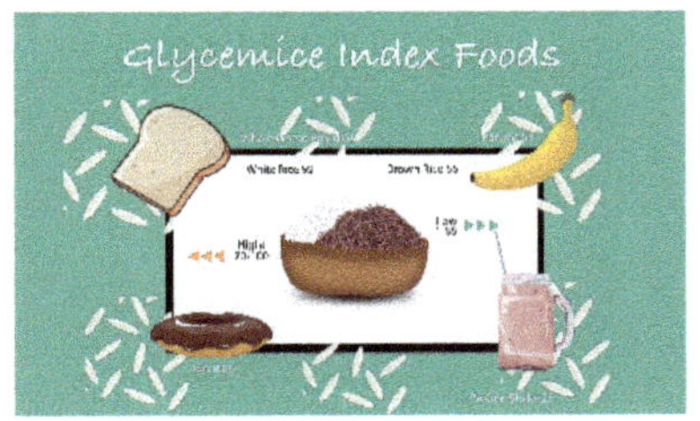

Meal GI = [(GI x amount of carbohydrate) Food A + (GI x amount of carbohydrate) Food B +...]/Total amount of available carbohydrate

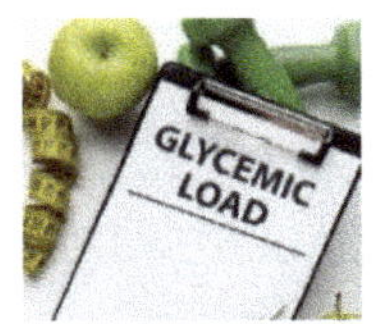

On the other hand, glycaemic load (GL) considers the amount of carbohydrates in a portion of food and how quickly it increases blood glucose levels.[10]

GL = GI x carbohydrate/100

For example, the GL of a slice of whole-grain bread= GI of bread (45) x carbohydrate content (18)/100

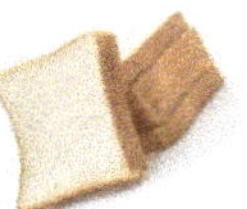

	GI	GL
Low	≤55	≤10
Medium	56–69	11–19
High	≥70	≥20

Decoding Food Labels

If you consume pre-packed foods, decoding the label information is paramount. Food labels provide us with vital information, such as the ingredients, nutrients contained, and how much they contribute to an average adult's energy requirements.[12]

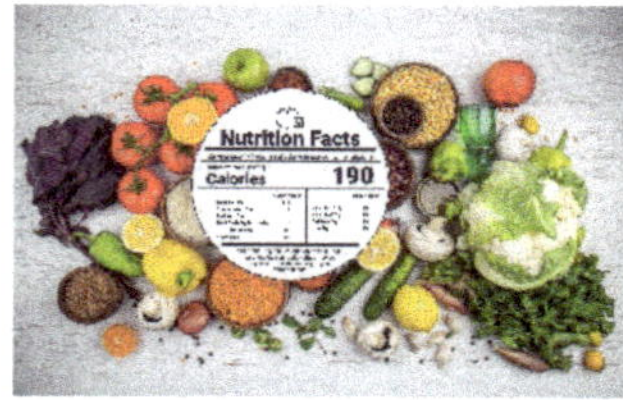

The ingredients are listed in descending order, with the highest-quantity ingredient listed first. So, if you see sugar at the top of the list, it's a good idea to ditch the food item.[12]

The traffic light system, while voluntary, offers a glance at the ingredients. The label has calories included in the food item and also color to indicate whether the food is high (red), medium (amber), and low (green) in salt, sugar, fat, and saturated fat.[12]

Each Serving Contains:

Calories	Sugars	Fat	Saturates	Salt
218	6.3g	3.2g	1.4g	0.5g
11%	7%	5%	7%	8%

Nutrition facts: This is the first place to start while scanning a food label. It provides information like serving size and number of servings in that package. This is important, as the serving size is related to the amount of nutrients and calories consumed.

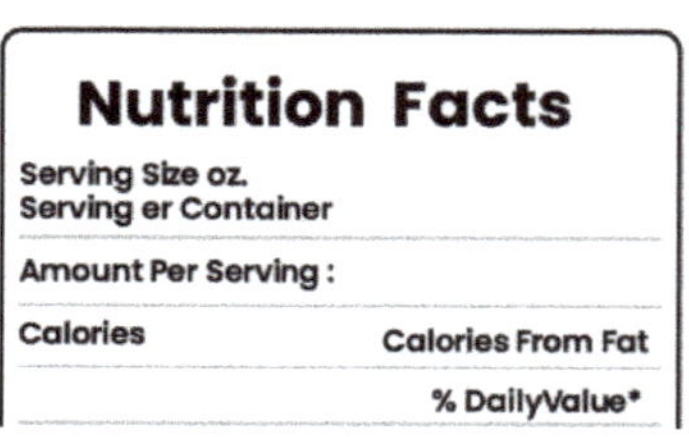

Calories: This provides a measure of energy you will consume from a serving of the food item. Here is a general guide to calories:[13]

Total Fat	%
Saturated Fat	%
Trans Fat	%
Cholesterol	%
Sodium	%
Total Carbohydrate	%
Dietary Fiber	%
Sugars	%
Protein	%

- 40 calories – Low
- 100 calories – Moderate
- 400 calories – High

Nutrients: This shows essential nutrients and separates them into two groups.

First group – Avoid the nutrients mentioned in the image on your left. Too much trans-fat, saturated fat, sodium, or cholesterol may increase your risk of high blood pressure or heart disease.

Second group – Get enough of the nutrients mentioned in the image to your right. They improve your health, aid digestion, and lower the risk of heart disease.[13]

Dietary fiber	g	%
Vitamin D	mcg	%
Calcium	mg	%
Iron	mg	%
Potassium	mg	%

% daily value (%DV): This indicates the quantity of a nutrient in one serving. The %DV is the percentage of the daily value that is recommended for a healthy person of four years and above for each nutrient in a single serving of the food item. You can use %DV to compare food products that are rich in nutrients and that you want to get more of.[13]

Nutribyte
%DV of 5% or lower indicates low nutrient content, whereas a value of 20% or more

Footnote: Most of the % daily values are provided according to a 2000-calorie diet. Your daily values may be lower or higher depending on your calorie needs.[13]

Key Takeaways

- Gestational diabetes is a common condition affecting almost 3%–5% of all pregnancies.
- Monitoring blood glucose levels; exercise; and dietary modifications (and medications in some case) help to ensure a healthy pregnancy.
- Always check food labels before consuming pre-packed foods.

Decode This Food Code

Time to fish out the Sherlock in you! Check if you can decipher this food label before your next grocery shopping spree.

a. How many servings does this packet of food provide?

b. Each serving of this food item contains 10 g of sugar. True/False

c. If you were to eat the entire packet, how many calories would you consume?

d. Saturated fat intake must be 20g/day (for a 2000 kcal diet). How much-saturated fat does one serving of this food item provide you with?

e. One packet of food provides 15 g of protein. True/false

f. How much percentage of your daily value for carbohydrate intake do two servings of this food item cover?

Nutrition Facts

Serving Size 10 oz.
Serving Per Container 5

Amount Per Serving

Calories 200	Calories From Fat 200
	% Daily value*
Total Fat 10 g	35%
Saturated Fat 1.5g	11%
Trans Fat 0.0 g	
Cholesterol 0 mg	1%
Sodium 210 mg	15%
Total Carbohydrate 15 g	3%
Dietary Fiber 2 g	3%
Sugars 3 g	
Protein 30 g	

Vitamin A	3%	Vitamin C	3%
Calcium	6%	Iron	6%

*Percent Daily values are based on a 2000 calorie diet. Your daily values may be higher or lewer depending on you calorie needs.

	Calories	2500	1500
Total Fat	Less Than	50g	25g
Saturated Fat	Less Than	55g	15g
Cholesterol	Less Than	35mg	15mg
Sodium	Less Than	15mg	50mg
Total Carbohydrate		300g	350g
Dietary Fieber	Less Than	20g	40g

Calories per gram
Fat 7 Carbohydrate 8 Protein 6

g. Does this food item contain cholesterol? Yes/No

Answers:

a. 12 servings
b. True
c. 1200 kcal (100 kcal per serving x 12 servings)
d. 3 g saturated fat
e. False, 12 g (1 g protein per serving x 12 servings)
f. 8% (4% DV per serving x 2 servings)
g. No

References

1. Plows JF, Stanley JL, Baker PN, *et al.* The pathophysiology of gestational diabetes mellitus. *Int J Mol Sci.* 2018;19(11):3342.
2. Gestational Diabetes. Available at: https://www.diabetes.co.uk/gestational-diabetes.html. It was accessed on 26 August 2019.
3. Kampmann U, Madsen LR, Skajaa GO, *et al.* Gestational diabetes: A clinical update. *World J Diabetes.* 2015;6(8):1065–1072.
4. Duman NB. Frequency of gestational diabetes mellitus and the associated risk factors. *Pak J Med Sci.* 2015;31(1):194–197.
5. NHS. Gestational diabetes – overview. Available at: https://www.nhs.uk/conditions/gestational-diabetes/. Accessed on 26 August 2019.
6. World Health Organization. Diagnostic criteria and classification of hyperglycemia first detected in pregnancy. Available at: https://www.ncbi.nlm.nih.gov/books/NBK169024/pdf/Bookshelf_NBK169024.pdf. Accessed on 26 August 2019.
7. Mayo Clinic. Gestational diabetes. Available at: https://www.mayoclinic.org/diseases-conditions/gestational-diabetes/diagnosis-treatment/drc-20355345. Accessed on 26 August 2019.

8. Gestational diabetes mellitus: Glycemic control and maternal prognosis. Available at: https://www.uptodate.com/contents/gestational-diabetes-mellitus-glycemic-control-and-maternal-prognosis#H1918741541. Accessed on: 26 August 2019.
9. Water and Diabetes. Available at https://www.diabetes.co.uk/food/water-and-diabetes.html Accessed on 26 August 2019.
10. Glycemic load. Available at: https://www.diabetes.co.uk/diet/glycemic-load.html. It was accessed on 26 August 2019.
11. Glycemic Index and Glycemic Load. Available at: https://lpi.oregonstate.edu/mic/food-beverages/glycemic-index-glycemic-load. Accessed on 26 August 2019.
12. It is understanding food labels. Available at: https://www.diabetes.org.uk/guide-to-diabetes/enjoy-food/food-shopping-for-diabetes/understanding-food-labels. Accessed on: 26 August 2019.
13. FDA. How to Understand and Use the Nutrition Facts Label. Available at: https://www.fda.gov/food/nutrition-education-resources-materials/how-understand-and-use-nutrition-facts-label. Accessed on: 26 August 2019.

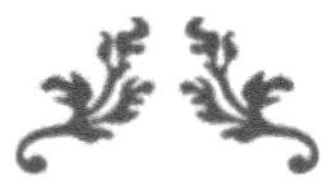

Scarlet was talking to her friend who was pregnant for the second time and was now nearing her eleventh week of pregnancy. They both were talking about precautions advised by their doctor. Her friend was worried about getting a blood test done. She was 30 during her last pregnancy and was diagnosed with anaemia during the second trimester. She used to be fatigued most of the time and had frequent headaches.

She was worried as she had several complications during her previous pregnancy due to anaemia. As she was nearing the second trimester, she had become more cautious. Listening to this, Scarlet decided to talk to her doctor. The doctor explained that not taking certain vitamin supplements increases the risk of anaemia, which can have a negative effect on both the mother and the baby. However, the good news is that it can be prevented and even treated by following an appropriate diet and consuming supplements as advised by the doctor.

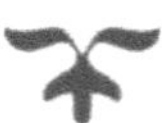

Chapter 9: Anaemia During Pregnancy

Anaemia is defined as a lower–than–average level of hemoglobin, the iron-imbued pigment in the red blood cells, which is responsible for carrying oxygen from the lungs to other cells of the body.[1,2]

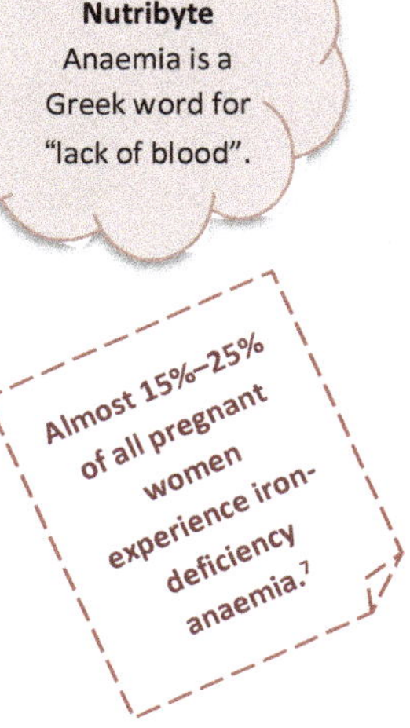

Various studies have shown that anaemia is one of the most common causes of preventable disorders in pregnancy. According to the World Health Organization, nearly 40% of pregnant women are anaemic worldwide.[1,2]

A woman's body goes through various changes during pregnancy. The blood

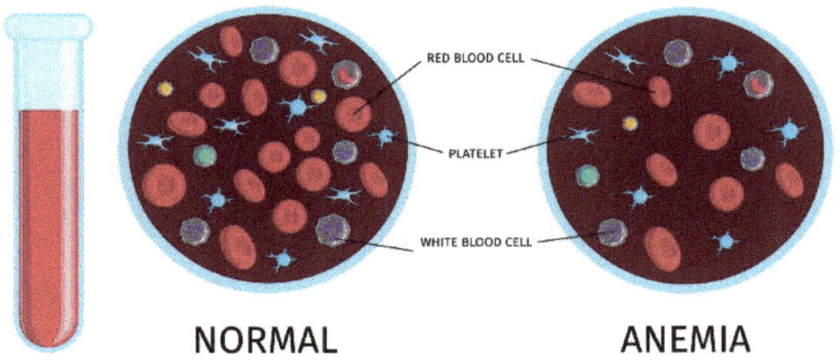

supply of the mother's body increases by 20% -30 %, which, in

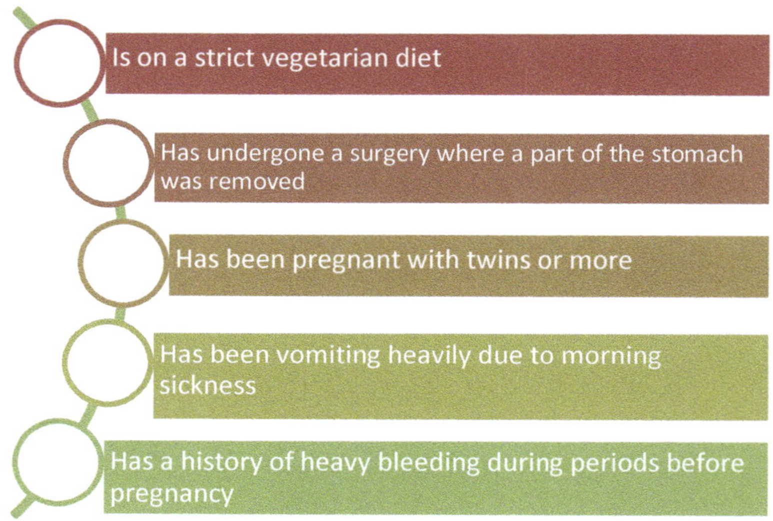

turn, increases the body's iron and vitamin requirements to make haemoglobin. If there is a lack of adequate nutrients, such as iron, folate, and vitamin B12, the body cannot produce sufficient haemoglobin, giving rise to anaemia.[1] The most common type of anaemia is iron-deficiency anaemia, where your body can't match its need for iron and, thus, low levels of haemoglobin.[3]

Mild anaemia is normal during pregnancy due to an increased blood volume. Severe anaemia, on the other hand, can pose a serious risk to the infant.[1]

Risk factors

Not all expecting mothers are anaemic. However, certain factors can lead to anaemia. A pregnant woman can become anaemic if she:[1,3]

In many cases, anaemia can be termed "silent" as no visible symptoms exist. In the remaining cases, fatigue, breathlessness, and drowsiness are commonly observed. Other symptoms of anaemia are given in figure below:[3,5]

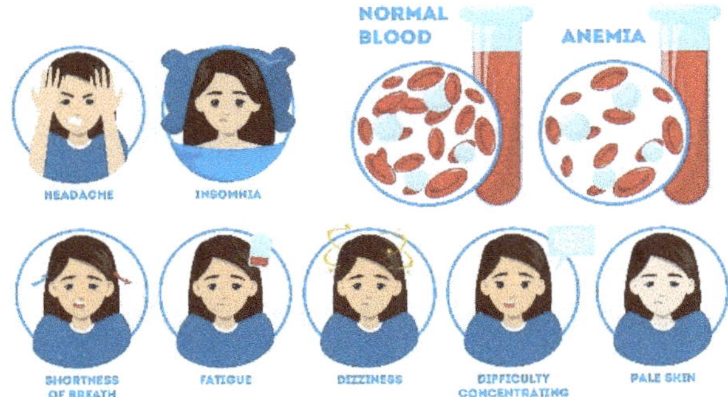

Causes of Anaemia: From Iron to Folate

The deficiency of various nutrients can lead to anaemia during pregnancy, and iron is one of them.[3] As mentioned earlier, iron is an essential constituent of haemoglobin. Low iron levels in the blood result in low haemoglobin levels and thus cause anaemia.[1,2] Iron deficiency anaemia can be caused by a low intake of iron-rich foods and foods that promote its absorption or an excess intake of foods that inhibit it.[6] The requirement of iron throughout gestation could be met easily by a continued increase in iron absorption rate. The irony about the iron requirement is that it varies during each trimester.[8]

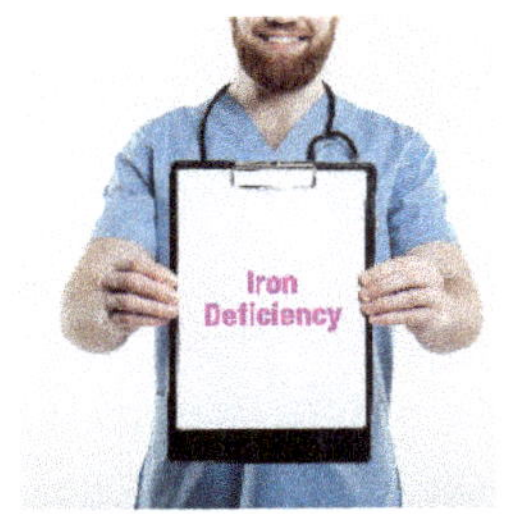

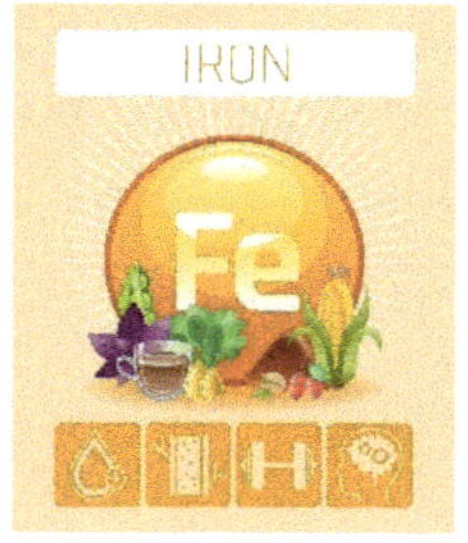

Iron requirement during the first trimester is low due to the cessation of menstruation. During the second trimester, the iron requirement increases, continuing throughout the rest of the pregnancy. Iron requirement ranges from 0.8 mg/day in the first trimester to 7.5 mg/day in the third trimester. Here is a list of the total iron requirement throughout gestation for different functions happening during pregnancy:[2,8]

Condition	Iron requirement
Development of the foetus	270 mg
Development of the placenta	80 mg
Delivery	250 mg
Increased blood requirement	450 mg
Basal loss	240 mg
Total Iron requirement	1040 mg

Vitamin B_{12} is vital for the production of healthy red blood cells. Vitamin B_{12} deficiency results in abnormal and fewer red blood cells, resulting in anaemia. Vitamin B_{12}-deficiency anaemia can cause preterm labour and neural tube defects.[6]

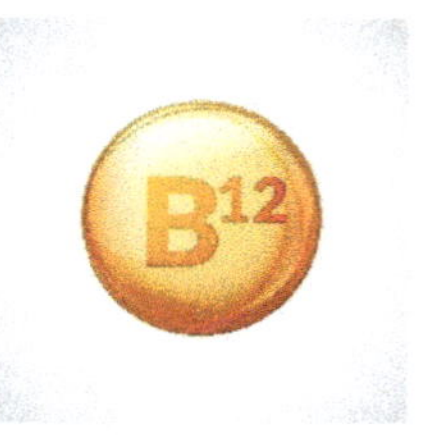

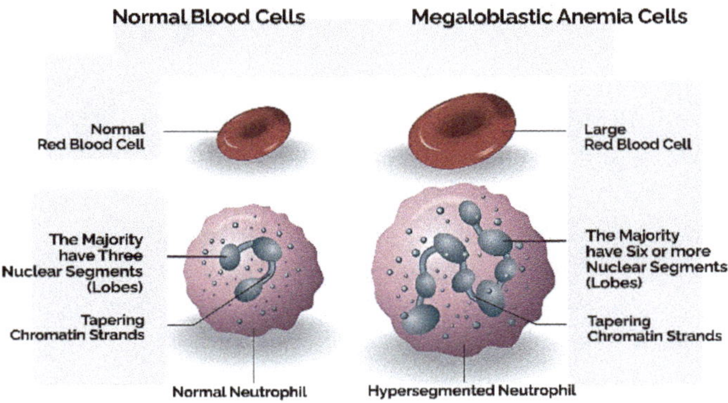

Folate, a type of vitamin B, produces new cells, including red blood cells. During pregnancy, the requirement for folate increases, and when this is not met through the diet, it can cause folate-deficiency anaemia. Folate deficiency can result in congenital disabilities like spina bifida (a defect where the spinal cord does not usually form).[6] In folate-deficiency anaemia, the red blood cells are more significant due to abnormal cell synthesis and are thus known as megaloblasts. This type of anaemia is known as megaloblastic anaemia. The symptoms of megaloblastic anaemia are similar to that of other anaemias.[9]

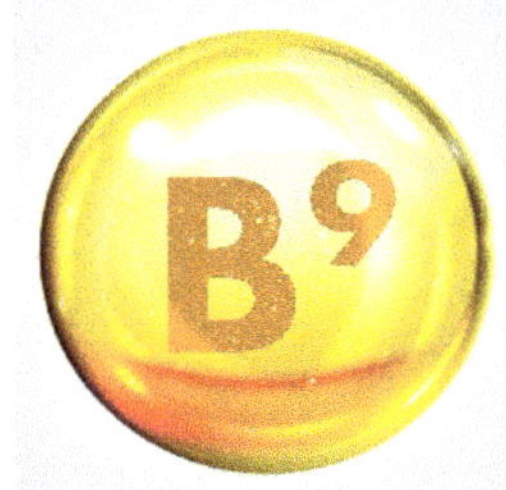

Ignorance is not bliss; spread the word, please!

Your doctor will test your blood for anaemia during your first prenatal visit and again later during various stages of your pregnancy, especially if you are at risk or have symptoms of anaemia. The haemoglobin level is the crucial determiner of anaemia.

A pregnant woman is said to be anaemic if her haemoglobin level is less than 11.0 gm/dL. A level below 4.0 gm/dL is defined as severe anaemia by the World Health Organization as it increases the maternal risk of congestive heart failure and death.[6]

Your doctor may also advise investigations that help determine the cause of anaemia. Some of them are as follows:[6]

- Serum iron levels
- Serum ferritin levels
- Total iron-binding capacity
- Vitamin B_{12} levels
- Folate levels

A healthy pregnancy is in your hands.

Maintaining your health, as well as your baby's, requires several nutrients. As anaemia is a result of nutrition deficiency, it can increase the risk of the following conditions:[10]

- Bleeding during pregnancy
- Excessive vomiting or hyperemesis gravidarum
- Gestational diabetes
- High blood pressure and protein in the urine, also known as preeclampsia,
- Intrauterine growth restriction (the baby does not grow in the womb as expected)
- Abnormal placement of the placenta
- Congenital anomalies

Eat Right and Beat Anaemia!

Consuming iron-rich foods can help prevent as well as manage iron-deficiency anaemia.

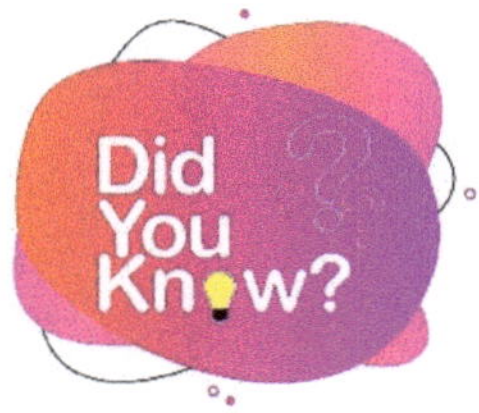

Two forms of dietary iron are haem iron and nonhaem iron.

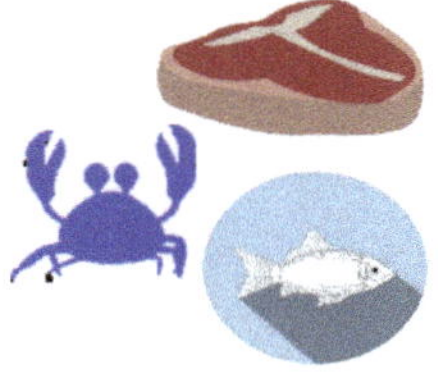

Haem iron is present in the haemoglobin and the myoglobin (a protein found in muscle tissue). It has a high bio-availability and is easily absorbed. It is mainly found in meat, fish, and seafood.[2]

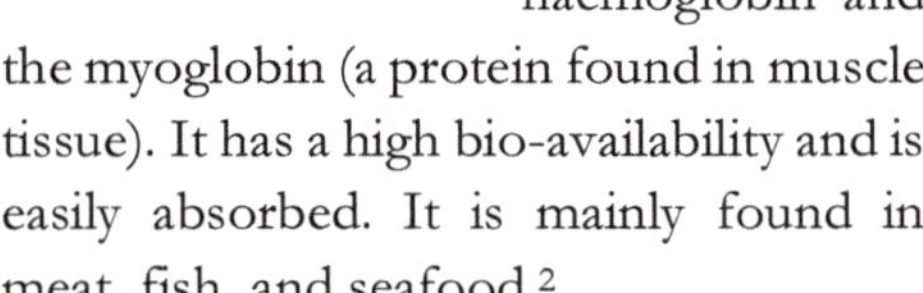

Nonhaem iron is most abundant in the vegetarian diet. It is mainly found in an oxidized form that is reduced by an enzyme in the cells lining the intestine. It has a lower bioavailability and is not absorbed easily. It is found in corn, wheat, barley, and legumes. It is also present in iron-fortified foods like bread, pasta, and dairy products.[2]

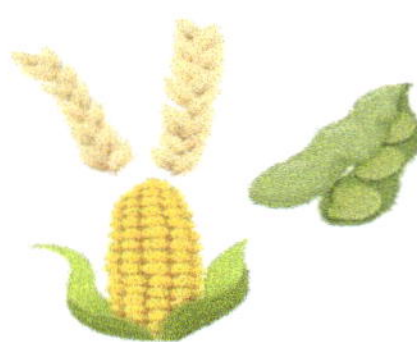

Factors affecting iron absorption: The absorption of nonhaem iron is influenced by various food items. The image below represents food items that maximize and inhibit non-haem iron absorption, respectively.[2]

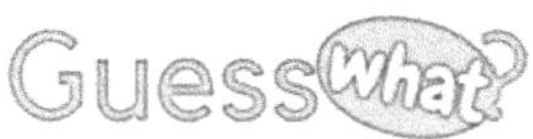

The helpers and the inhibitors play an important role in preventing anaemia.

Take the following precautions and prevent anaemia:[12]

Include the following helpers in your diet:

- ✓ Beef, chicken, and lamb meat as these increase the absorption of nonhaem iron
- ✓ Fruits and honey instead of sugar as it is seen to improve iron absorption
- ✓ Carotenoids, yellow to red pigment, found in certain foods, such as carrots, oranges, and peaches, which help in the absorption of iron
- ✓ Consuming 100 mg of ascorbic acid can increase iron absorption from a specific meal by 4.14 times. Food rich in ascorbic acid are oranges, pineapples, and berries.

Limit intake of the following inhibitors:

- ✗ Calcium, in the amount of 300–600 mg, can inhibit the absorption of both, haem and nonhaem iron. A cup of skimmed milk contains approximately 300 mg of calcium. When calcium is recommended, it is usually advised to be taken at bedtime.
- ✗ Phosvitin, a protein in eggs, prevents absorption of iron. It is seen that consuming a boiled egg can reduce iron absorption of a meal by 28%.
- ✗ Phytate, a compound present in food items, such as sesame and almonds can lower iron absorption by 50 %–65%.
- ✗ Tea and coffee can be taken between the meals instead of taking them along with the meals as phytates in them prevent the absorption of iron.

Foods with high iron content

Here is a list of iron-rich foods and the quantity required to get a specific amount of iron:[11]

Foods that provide 0.5–1.5 mg of iron

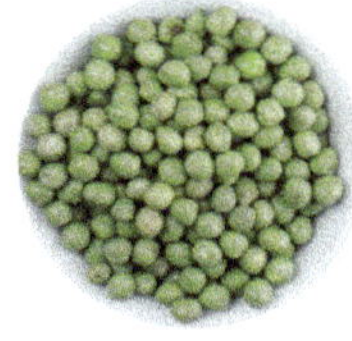

Half cup of green peas

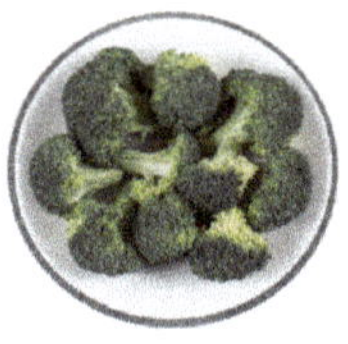

Half cup of broccoli

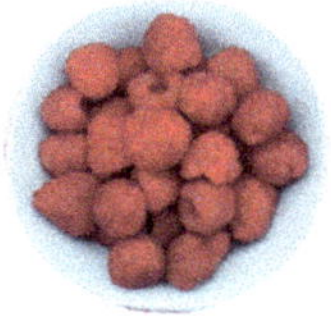

One cup of raspberries

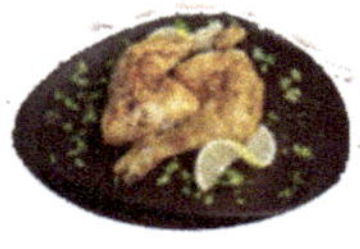

3 oz of chicken

Foods that provide 1.6–3 mg of iron

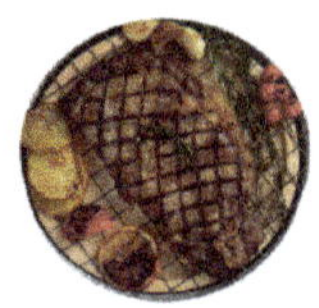

3 oz of roasted beef

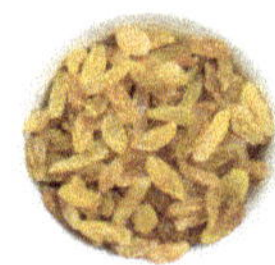

Half cup of raisins

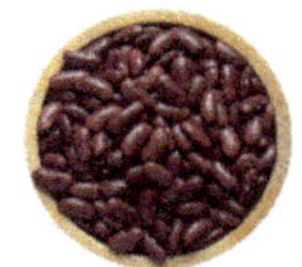

Half cup of kidney beans

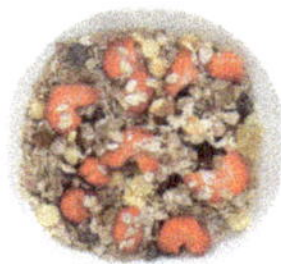

One cup of cooked oatmeal

Foods that provide 3-12 mg of iron

Four large or six medium clams
Nine small oysters

Half cup of cooked spinach

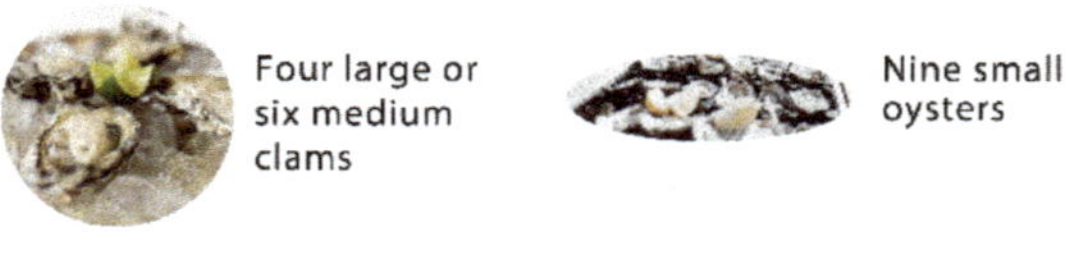

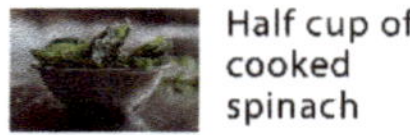

Some tips to prevent anaemia:

- Eat iron-rich food, such as meat, fish, and vegetables.
- Consume foods rich in folic acid, such as dried beans, orange juice, green leafy vegetables, and wheat germ.
- Cooking in cast iron vessels can add up to 80% more iron to your meal.[1]

To supplement or not!

The Institute of Medicine (US) Committee recommends iron supplementation at 30 mg/day after 12 weeks of pregnancy to prevent iron-deficiency anaemia. A dose of 60–120 mg of iron is recommended if your blood tests indicate anaemia at any stage of gestation. This dose is usually lowered to 30 mg/day when blood tests show that your haemoglobin levels are now within the normal range for the stage of pregnancy.[2]

Although iron supplements are safe, they can cause certain side effects. If you experience any of the below-mentioned symptoms, you should contact your doctor:[2]

- Heartburn
- Upper abdominal discomfort
- Nausea
- Diarrhea
- Constipation

It is always recommended to consult your physician before starting any supplement, especially during pregnancy.

Psssstttt.......

Anaemia can cause some people to chew ice. Yes, you heard it right. Anaemia can cause PICA, a medical term used for the compulsion to chew substances devoid of nutrition, such as clay, ice, and paper. It is a more distinctive symptom of iron-deficiency anaemia.[13]

Key Takeaways

- Iron-deficiency anaemia is the most common type of anaemia that occurs during pregnancy.
- Your diet and certain health conditions before or during pregnancy can increase your risk of developing anaemia.
- Anaemia during pregnancy can lead to complications, such as hypertension and diabetes
- Consuming the right diet and taking nutritional supplements as advised by your doctor can prevent the risk of complications.

It is time for a nutritional quiz to put your knowledge about "the helpers" and "the inhibitors" to the test.

Group the following items as helpers and inhibitors:

1. Eggs
2. Meat
3. Fruits
4. Calcium
5. Walnuts
6. Coffee
7. Carrots
8. Oranges

Helpers: 2,3,7, and 8

Inhibitors: 1,4,5, and 6

References

47. American Society of Hematology. Anaemia and Pregnancy. Available at: https://www.hematology.org/Patients/Anaemia/Pregnancy.aspx. Accessed on 30 August 2019.

48. Institute of Medicine (US) Committee on Nutritional Status During Pregnancy and Lactation. Iron Nutrition During Pregnancy. Nutrition During Pregnancy. Available at: https://www.ncbi.nlm.nih.gov/books/NBK235217/. Accessed on 30 August 2019.

49. Anaemia in pregnancy. Available at: https://www.cedars-sinai.org/health-library/diseases-and-conditions/a/anaemia-in-pregnancy.html. Accessed on 30 August 2019.

50. Your guide to anaemia. Available at: https://www.nhlbi.nih.gov/files/docs/public/blood/anaemia-yg.pdf. Accessed on 30 August 2019.

51. The FASEB journal. Association Between Anaemia Subtypes and Insomnia Symptoms in Community-Dwelling Older Adults. Available at: https://www.fasebj.org/doi/abs/10.1096/fasebj.29.1_supplement.392.7. Accessed on 30 August 2019.

52. National Health Portal of India. Anaemia during pregnancy (Maternal anaemia). Available at: https://www.nhp.gov.in/disease/gynaecology-and-obstetrics/anaemia-during-pregnancy-maternal-anaemia. Accessed on: 30 August 2019.

53. American Pregnancy Association. Anaemia During Pregnancy. Available at: https://americanpregnancy.org/pregnancy-concerns/anaemia-during-pregnancy/. Accessed on 30 August 2019.

54. The American Journal of Clinical Nutrition. Iron requirements in pregnancy and strategies to meet them. Available at:

https://academic.oup.com/ajcn/article/72/1/257S/4729643 Accessed on: 30 August 2019.

55. MedlinePlus. Folate-deficiency anaemia. Available at https://medlineplus.gov/ency/article/000551.htm. Accessed on 30 August 2019.

56. Taner CE, Ekin A, Solmaz U, *et al.* Prevalence and risk factors of anaemia among pregnant women attending a high-volume tertiary care center for delivery. *J Turk Ger Gynecol Assoc.* 2015;16(4):231–236.

57. UCSH Health. Anaemia and pregnancy. Available at: https://www.ucsfhealth.org/education/anaemia_and_pregnancy/. Accessed on 30 August 2019.

58. Iron Disorders Institute. Available at: http://www.irondisorders.org/diet. Accessed on 30 August 2019.

59. American Society of Hematology. Iron-Deficiency Anaemia. Available at: https://www.hematology.org/Patients/Anaemia/Iron-Deficiency.aspx. Accessed on 30 August 2019.

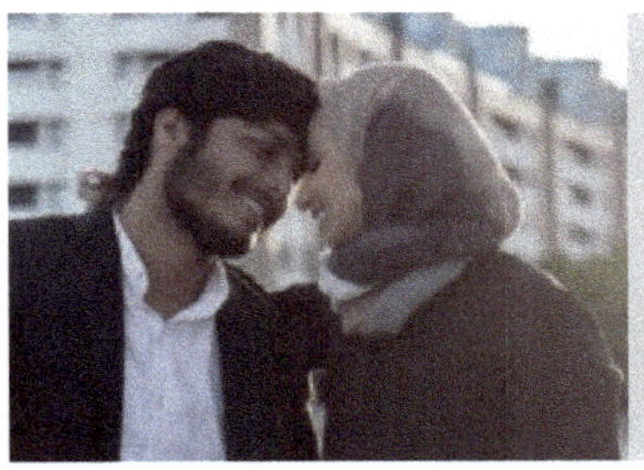

Chapter 10 Impact of Nutrition on Preterm Birth and Miscarriage

An estimated about 1 in 8 pregnancies will end in miscarriage

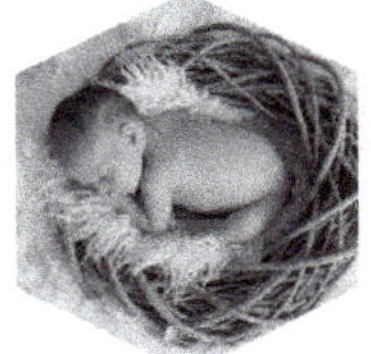

Every year, an estimated 15 million babies are born too early

Miscarriage: Nutritional Status and Non-nutritive Substances

Miscarriage can be a devastating event that may have long-lasting repercussions. It can be both disappointing and frustrating to both parents. What is a miscarriage? A miscarriage is an unsuccessful outcome of pregnancy, wherein an embryo or foetus dies before the twentieth week of pregnancy. Various reasons could be cited for miscarriage, but, most often, the exact cause cannot be identified.[3,4] However, lifestyle factors such as malnutrition, smoking, drug use, excessive caffeine intake, and exposure to radiation or toxic substances have been associated with adverse pregnancy outcomes, including miscarriage. Among lifestyle factors, a woman's nutritional status plays a critical role in maintaining a healthy pregnancy. Malnutrition includes overweight, obesity, undernutrition, and micronutrient (vitamin or mineral) deficiency.

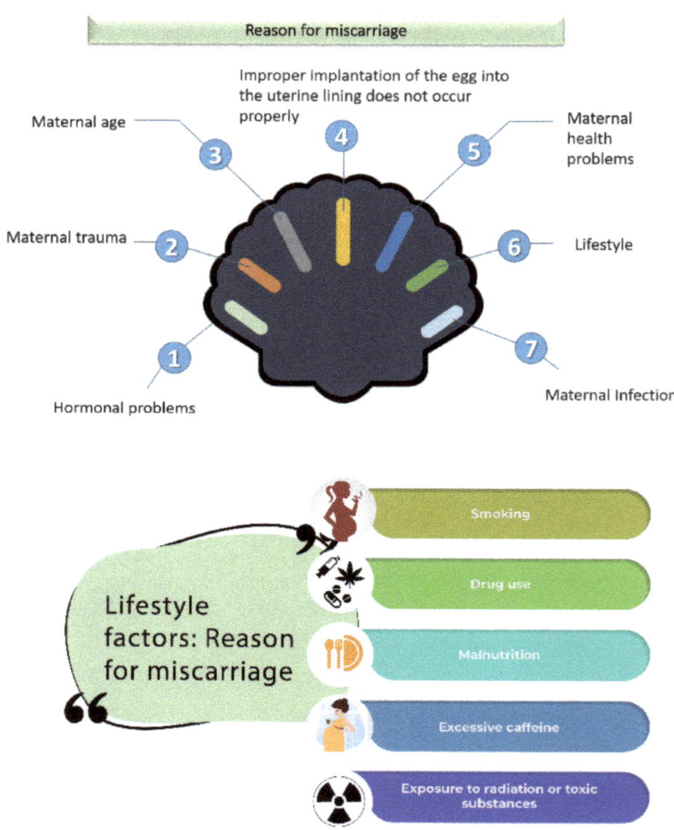

Overnutrition can lead to obesity, which has a major impact on female fertility; obesity is considered a cause of not only miscarriage but also conjugal infertility.[5] Obesity is associated with a considerably high risk of miscarriage. Data on obese women attending infertility clinics clearly show that such women have a lower number of mature oocytes (an immature ovum or egg cell), as well as oocytes with reduced diameter.[5] It is indeed challenging to help obese women conceive through *in vitro* fertilization (IVF) because embryos formed from the ova of overweight and obese women exhibit a lower potential for development after IVF.[5]

The chances of recurrent
pregnancy loss is 1.75
times in odese women

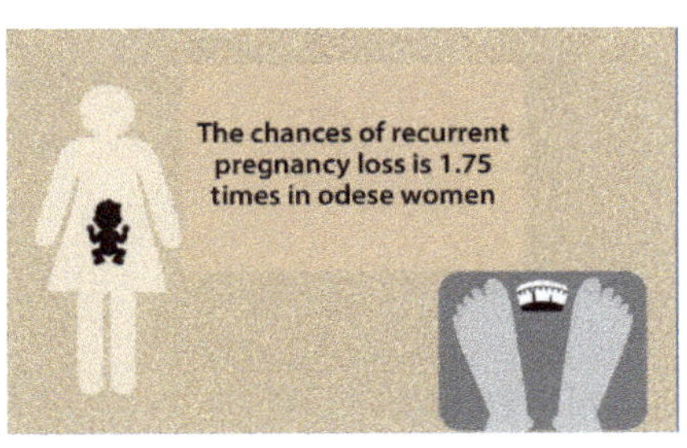

Poor maternal weight has also been associated with poor pregnancy outcomes, including low birth weight, birth asphyxia, anaemia, and increased perinatal mortality rates.[6] Underweight women face an increased risk of miscarriage, perhaps due to downregulation of hormones or as a direct consequence of undernutrition.[7] Leptin, which is primarily considered to affect appetite and weight regulation, is also known to positively affect reproductive health. Low serum leptin levels could be linked to spontaneous abortion, and women with a low body mass index have low leptin levels. Clinical evidence indicates that women suffering a spontaneous abortion have lower serum leptin in their first trimester compared to both pregnant and nonpregnant women.[7]

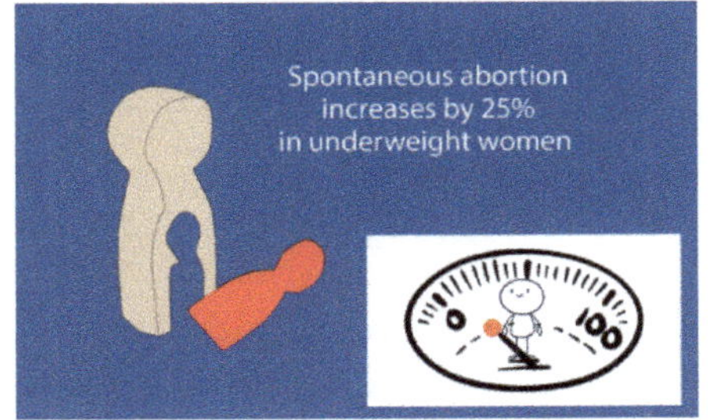

Drinking alcohol or smoking during pregnancy is not a healthy lifestyle choice, especially for women of reproductive age. Both increase the odds of pregnancy loss.[8]

Consuming even a small amount of alcohol during the first four months of pregnancy is likely to increase the risk of miscarriage.[8] Evidence strongly supports an association between alcohol consumption during pregnancy and miscarriage. Consuming two to four alcoholic drinks per week during pregnancy is related to miscarriage, and the risk is particularly high during the early (<10 weeks gestation) phase of pregnancy. The adverse effects of alcohol on the foetus or embryo are greatest when it is especially sensitive to environmental insults.[8]

Alcohol may
harm human
foetuses not
only when it is
abused but also
when taken in
moderation

There is no known safe amount or safe time of alcohol use during pregnancy or in the preconception phase.[9]

Smoking during pregnancy is directly linked to the risk of miscarriage. Exposure to second-hand smoke, too, increases the risk of miscarriage.[10]

Even if a woman has never smoked, there is a 20% risk of miscarriage if she has lived with two or more smokers as a child. There is a 14% higher risk of pregnancy loss among women exposed to second-hand smoke five or more times per week compared to women not exposed to it during childhood.[11]

Secondhand smoke exposure during pregnancy increased the risk of miscarriage by 11%

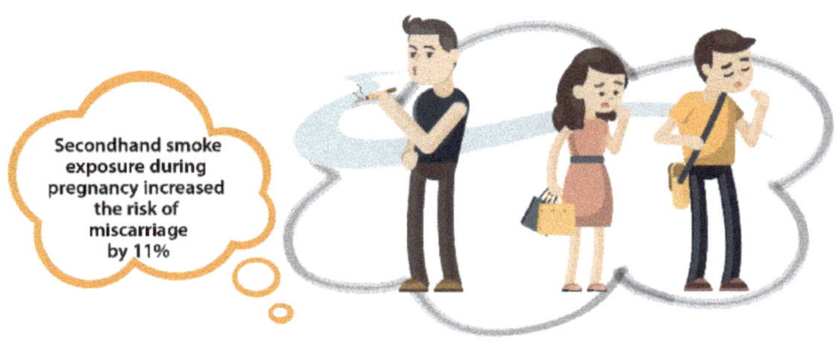

Role of Nutrition in Miscarriage

Diets with large amounts of red meat, high-fat dairy products, and simple carbohydrates are associated with high levels of immunological markers, which are typically observed in obese women with recurrent pregnancy loss.[5]

Women who consume a more pro-inflammatory diet have a higher risk of abortion compared with those who consume a more anti-inflammatory diet.[12]

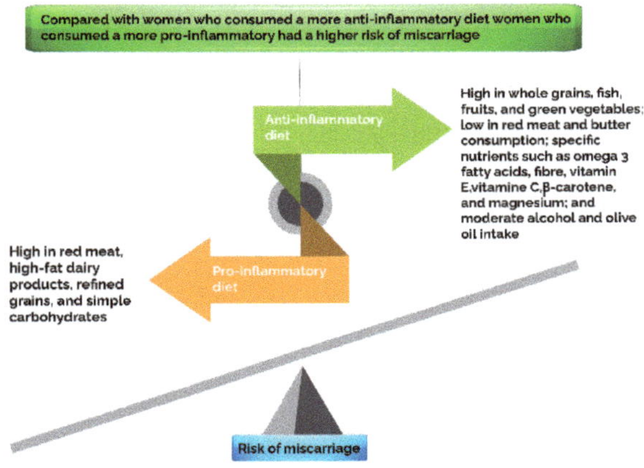

The lesser the consumption of green vegetables, fruit, milk, cheese, eggs, and fish, the greater the risk of spontaneous abortion. The chances of miscarriage are double and one-and-a-half times following the highest consumption of butter and oil, respectively. Women have a high risk of miscarriage if they consume alcohol and coffee during the preconception stage.[13]

A diet poor in micronutrients (carotenoids, folates, vitamins, and calcium) correlates to an increased risk of spontaneous abortion.[13]

Fish oil containing eicosapentaenoic acid (EPA) and docosahexaenoic acid (DHA) could prevent recurrent miscarriage, especially in women with a special medical condition known as antiphospholipid syndrome.[14]

Women consuming any fish oil stand a chance of lowering their risk of pregnancy loss by 20%. Women receiving DHA supplementation in the preconception stage or during pregnancy are five times less likely to experience pregnancy loss compared to those who do not receive DHA supplementation.[15]

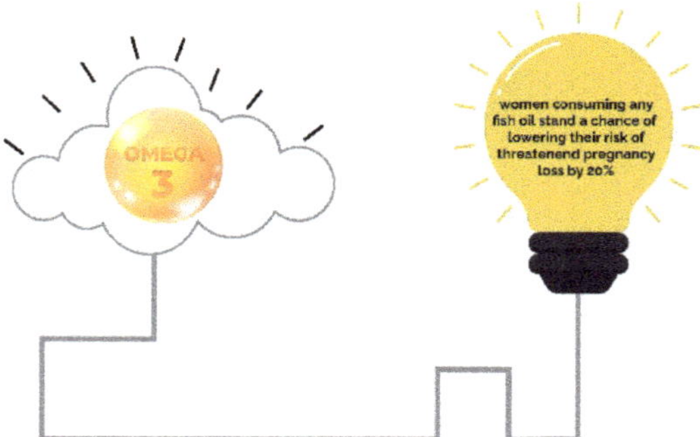

Inadequate intake of vitamin D has been linked to miscarriage, especially in women with prior miscarriage.[16]

Hence, it is prudent to believe that consuming a diet poor in vegetables, fruit, milk, and dairy products but rich in fats could increase the risk of spontaneous abortion.

Poor dietary intake of vitamins has been associated with an increased risk of miscarriage. Hence, vitamin supplementation before or in early pregnancy may help prevent miscarriage.[17]

Make a Healthy Choice to Keep Your Ongoing Pregnancy Healthy

Several factors can be attributed to adverse pregnancy outcomes, such as miscarriages or preterm delivery. A few simple steps can be taken to ensure a successful pregnancy. Be it before pregnancy or during pregnancy, women should.[3]

- Exercise regularly
- Eat healthily
- Manage stress
- Keep weight within healthy limits
- Take folic acid daily
- Quit smoking

Did You Know?

Alcohol and pregnancy: Even if your pregnancy is saved, your child may not escape from foetal alcohol spectrum disorders.

There is no known safe amount or safe time of alcohol consumption during pregnancy and in women of reproductive age. Foetal alcohol spectrum disorders refer to a group of conditions in a child whose mother consumed alcohol during pregnancy. Foetal alcohol spectrum disorders are associated with brain damage, which affects behavior and learning. It is also associated with growth problems.[18]

Depending on the nature of symptoms, foetal alcohol spectrum disorders could be described as foetal alcohol syndrome (FAS), alcohol-related neurodevelopmental disorders (ARNDs), alcohol-related birth defects (ARBDs), and neurobehavioural disorders associated with prenatal alcohol exposure.[18]

There is no cure for foetal alcohol spectrum disorders! Remember this before you consume alcohol.[18]

Role of Maternal Nutrition in Preterm Birth

Maternal nutrition during pregnancy is a key determinant of pregnancy outcomes, and it plays an important role in providing the necessary nutrients for foetal growth.

Impact of Maternal Nutrition on Preterm Delivery

An imbalance in maternal nutrition may increase the risk of preterm birth, which in turn could have a lifelong impact on the health of a preterm infant. Preterm infants may have to live with compromised physical growth, deficits in executive function, and behavioral, attention, and learning problems.[19]

An assessment of the diets of mothers of preterm infants revealed that the former had lower total energy and fat intake compared to women who delivered at term. In addition, mothers delivering preterm babies had higher intakes of retinol but lower intakes of niacin, vitamin E, copper, and magnesium compared to women who delivered at term. Also, among mothers delivering preterm babies, intakes of vitamin A, calcium, and iron were much lower than the Dietary Reference Intakes.[19]

Significance of Maternal Nutrition in Improving Pregnancy Outcomes

Maternal consumption of fruits, root vegetables, cabbages, potatoes, oatmeal porridge, whole grains, wild fish, game, berries, milk, and water lowers the risk of spontaneous preterm delivery.[20]

A diet ensuring adequate micronutrient intake from green leafy vegetables, fruits, whole-grain breads/cereals, oily fish, and eggs is likely to positively influence the development of the placenta. A micronutrient-rich diet could decrease the risk of developing adverse pathologies that favor premature delivery.[20]

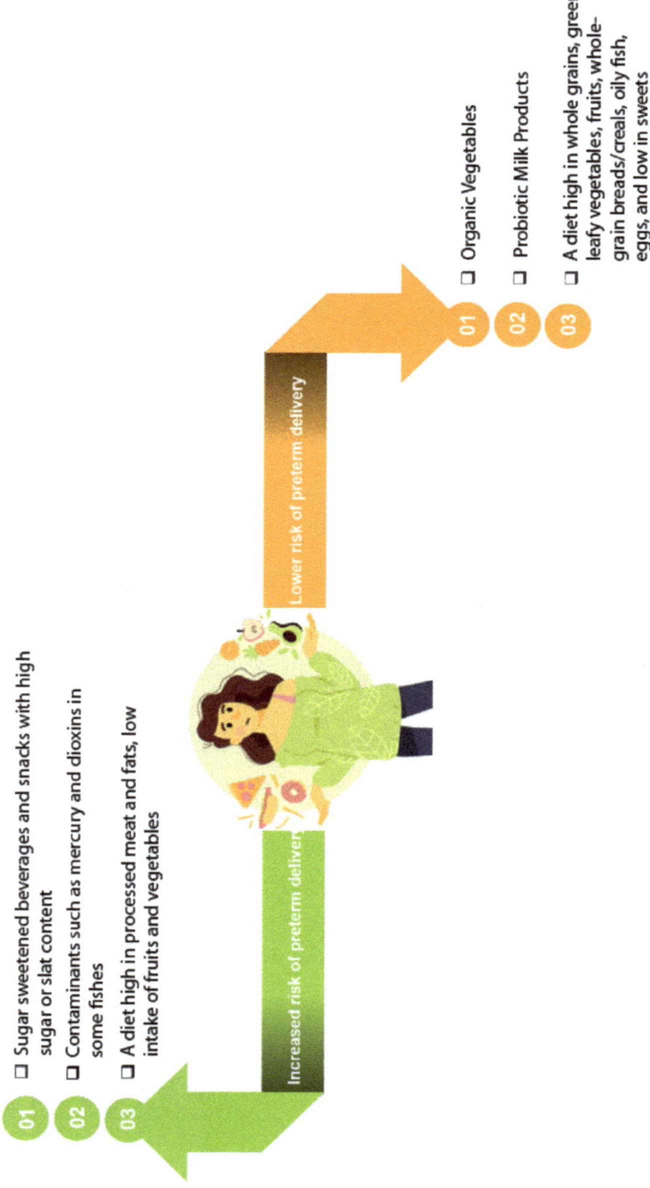
01 Sugar sweetened beverages and snacks with high sugar or slat content
02 Contaminants such as mercury and dioxins in some fishes
03 A diet high in processed meat and fats, low intake of fruits and vegetables
Increased risk of preterm deliver
Lower risk of preterm delivery
01 Organic Vegetables
02 Probiotic Milk Products
03 A diet high in whole grains, green leafy vegetables, fruits, whole-grain breads/creals, oily fish, eggs, and low in sweets

A diet consisting of raw and cooked vegetables, salad, onion, garlic, fruit, berries, nuts, vegetable oils, whole-grain cereals, poultry, and fiber-rich bread significantly reduces the risk of preterm delivery by 12%.[20]

Benefits of Nutrient Supplementation During Pregnancy

Preterm delivery might be prevented if the maternal diet comprises vegetables, fruit, and berries that are rich in antioxidants and vitamins, which can reduce both systemic and local inflammation.[21]

It has been hypothesized that increased maternal intake of omega-3 fatty acids can offset the prostaglandin pathway associated with inflammation and preterm birth. Nonconsumption of fish could reduce the duration of pregnancy. Evidence indicates that supplementation with omega-3 fatty acids could considerably reduce the risk of preterm (<37 gestational weeks) and early preterm (<34 gestation weeks) delivery.[22]

Folic acid status, before conception or in early pregnancy, could avert the risk of preterm delivery. This protective effect could be ensured if folic acid is consumed for at least one year before conception.[22]

Iron plays a significant role in influencing pregnancy outcomes, although the evidence is less convincing. Iron supplementation may prolong the duration of pregnancy.[22]

Mild to–moderate zinc deficiency is a frequent finding in pregnant women, and zinc supplementation during pregnancy could help in preventing preterm birth by 14%.[23]

High-dose calcium supplementation ($\geq$1 g/day) is projected to reduce the risk of preterm delivery, especially in pregnant women consuming low-calcium diets.[24]

Keeping in view the importance of diet and pregnancy outcomes such as loss of pregnancy and preterm delivery, pregnant women must take measures to improve the quality of their diet.

Key Takeaways

- Malnutrition is a lifestyle factor strongly related to reduced reproductive capacity.
- Obesity is an independent risk factor for early pregnancy loss.
- Obese and underweight women have an increased risk of miscarriage.
- Exposure to second-hand smoke during childhood is associated with a higher risk of pregnancy loss.
- A diet poor in vegetables, fruit, milk, and dairy products, but rich in fats, could increase the risk of spontaneous abortion.
- An imbalance in maternal nutrition may increase the risk of preterm birth.
- Preterm delivery might be prevented by ensuring the maternal diet comprises vegetables, fruit, and berries rich in antioxidants and vitamins, which can reduce both systemic and local inflammation.

Wander Word: Impact of Nutrition on Preterm Birth and Miscarriage

Tickle your brain to find the answers!

One among the many lifestyle causes for pregnancy loss.

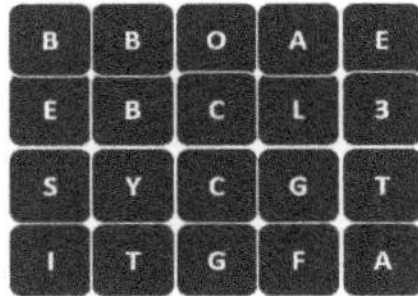

Obesity

One the key maternal supplementation that can offset prostaglandin pathway associated with inflammation and preterm birth.

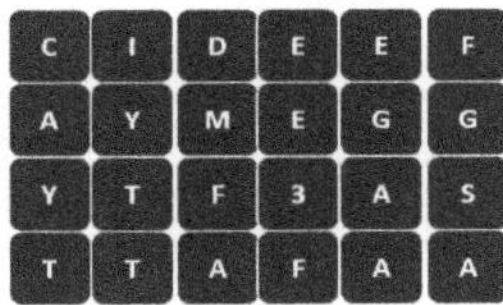

omega 3 fatty acids

Women can have a higher chance of miscarriage following its consumption in the preconception stage

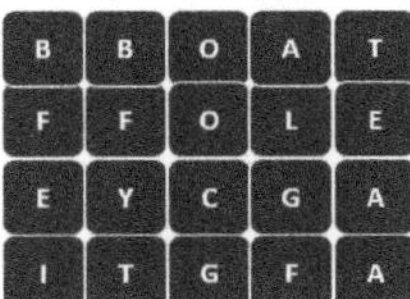

Coffee

A conditions in a child, whose mother had had consumed excess alcohol during pregnancy

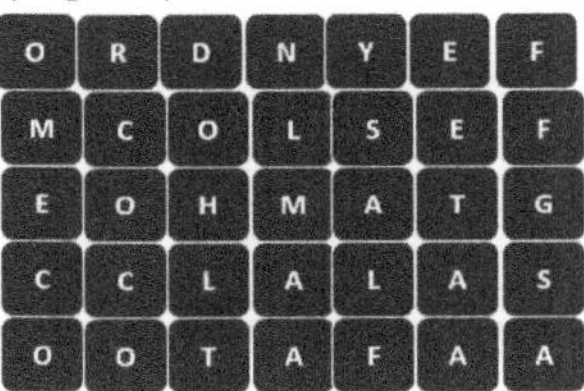

Fetal alcohol syndrome

An unsuccessful outcome of pregnancy wherein an embryo or fetus dies before the twentieth week of pregnancy

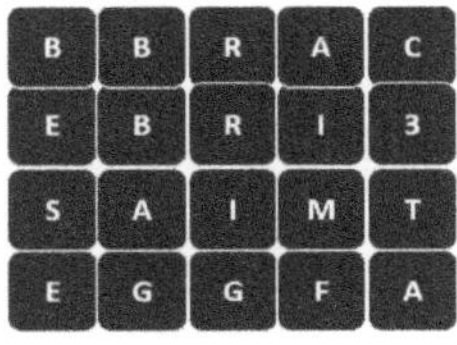

Miscarriage

References

1. NHS. Miscarriage. Available from: https://www.nhs.uk/conditions/miscarriage/. Accessed on: 7 September 2019.
2. Preterm birth. Available from: who. Int/en/news-room/fact-sheets/detail/preterm-birth. Accessed on: 7 September 2019.
3. American Pregnancy Association. Miscarriage. Available at: https://americanpregnancy.org/pregnancy-complications/miscarriage/. Accessed on: 4 September 2019.
4. Griebel CP, Halvorsen J, Golemon TB, *et al.* Management of spontaneous abortion. *I am a Fam Physician.* 2005;72(7):1243–1250.
5. Cavalcante MB, Sarno M, Peixoto AB, *et al.* Obesity and recurrent miscarriage: A systematic review and meta-analysis. *J Obstet Gynaecol Res.* 2010;45(1):30–38.
6. Sebire NJ, Jolly M, Harris J, *et al.* Is maternal underweight a risk factor for adverse pregnancy outcomes? A population-based study in London. *BJOG.* 2001;108(1):61–66.
7. Helgstrand S, Andersen A-M N. Maternal underweight and the risk of spontaneous abortion. *Acta Obstet Gynecol Scand.* 2005: 84: 1197–1201.
8. Avalos LA, Roberts SC, Kaskutas LA, *et al.* Volume and type of alcohol during early pregnancy and the risk of miscarriage. *Subst Use Misuse.* 2014;49(11):1437–1445.
9. CDC. Alcohol and Pregnancy Questions and Answers. Available at: https://www.cdc.gov/ncbddd/fasd/faqs.html. Accessed on: 7 Sep 2019
10. Pineles BL, Park E, Samet JM. Systematic review and meta-analysis of miscarriage and maternal exposure to tobacco smoke during pregnancy. *Am J Epidemiol.* 2014;179(7):807–823.

11. Yang S, Xu L, He Y, *et al.* Childhood secondhand smoke exposure and pregnancy loss in never smokers: The Guangzhou Biobank Cohort Study. *Tob Control.* 2017;26(6):697–702. doi:10.1136/tobaccocontrol-2016-053239.
12. Vahid F, Shivappa N, Hekmatdoost A, *et al.* Association between Maternal Dietary Inflammatory Index (DII) and abortion in Iranian women and validation of DII with serum concentration of inflammatory factors: a case-control study. *Appl Physiol Nutr Metab.* 2017;42(5):511–516.
13. Di Cintio E, Parazzini F, Chatenoud L, *et al.* Dietary factors and risk of spontaneous abortion. *Eur J Obstet Gynecol Reprod Biol.* 2001;95(1):132–136.
14. Rossi E, Costa M. Fish oil derivatives as a prophylaxis of recurrent miscarriage associated with antiphospholipid antibodies (APL): A pilot study. *Lupus.* 1993;2(5):319-23.
15. Tan TC, Neo GH, Malhotra R. Lifestyle risk factors associated with threatened miscarriage: A case-control study. *JFIV Reprod Med Genet.* 2014, 2:2 DOI: 10.4172/jfiv.1000123.
16. Andersen LB, Jørgensen JS, Jensen TK, *et al.* Vitamin D insufficiency is associated with an increased risk of first-trimester miscarriage in the Odense Child Cohort. *Am J Clin Nutr.* 2015;102:633–638
17. Balogun OO, da Silva Lopes K, Ota E, *et al.* Vitamin supplementation for preventing miscarriage. *Cochrane Database Syst Rev.* 2016, Issue 5. Art. No.: CD004073. DOI: 10.1002/14651858.CD004073.pub4.
18. CDC. Foetal alcohol syndrome. Available at: https://www.cdc.gov/ncbddd/fasd/facts.html. Accessed on: 10 Sep 2019.
19. Zhang Y, Zhou H, Perkins A, *et al.* Maternal dietary nutrient intake and its association with preterm birth: A case-control study in Beijing, China. *Nutrients.* 2017;9(3):221. doi:10.3390/nu9030221.

20. Cetin I, Laoreti A. The importance of maternal nutrition for health. *J Pediatr Neonat Individual Med.* 2015;4(2):e040220. doi: 10.7363/040220.
21. Englund-Ögge L, Brantsæter AL, Sengpiel V, *et al.* Maternal dietary patterns and preterm delivery: Results from a large prospective cohort study. *BMJ.* 2014;348:g1446.
22. Bloomfield FH. How is maternal nutrition related to preterm birth? *Ann Rev Nutrit.*2010;31:235–261.
23. Ota E, Mori R, Middleton P, *et al.* Zinc supplementation for improving pregnancy and infant outcomes. *Cochrane Database Syst Rev.* 2015, Issue 2. Art. No.: CD000230.DOI: 10.1002/14651858.CD000230.pub5
24. Hofmeyr GJ, Lawrie TA, Atallah ÁN, *et al.* Calcium supplementation during pregnancy for preventing hypertensive disorders and related problems. *Cochrane Database Syst Rev.* 2018 Oct 1;10:CD001059. doi: 10.1002/14651858.CD001059.pub5.

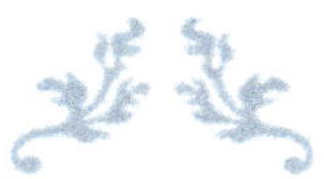

The rise of childhood obesity has placed the health of an entire generation at risk.

–Tom Vilsack

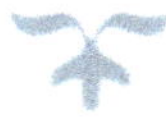

Chapter 11
Impact of Maternal Nutrition on Long-Term Health of Mother and Child

Today, we have unprecedented, easy access to junk food. The consumption of junk food is widely promoted; as a result, nutrition is affected – even during pregnancy. Recent times have witnessed an increased prevalence of chronic diseases. Various studies link hostile exposure in early life, especially those about nutrition, with chronic diseases. Developmental origins of health and disease (DOHaD) is a new field of study that aids in understanding the putative concepts and mechanisms that relate specific exposures in early life with the risk of developing chronic conditions in adulthood.[1] Perinatal undernutrition, as well as nutrient excess, can predispose a child to various conditions.[1] Want to understand why exactly this happens? Read on to find out.

Epigenetics – It's Not Just Genes That Make Us

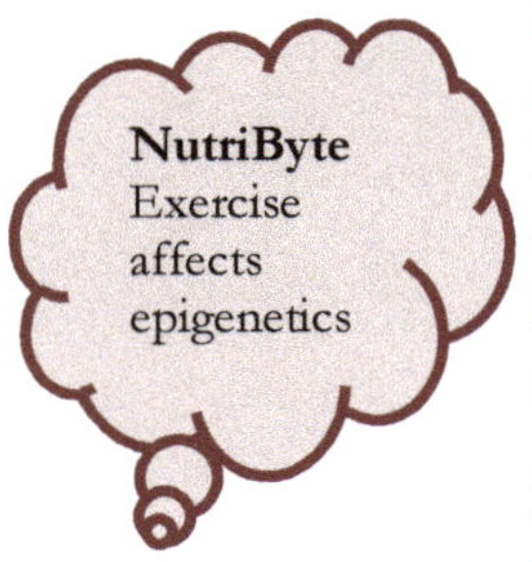

Epigenetics is a term used to refer to all modifications to genes, except in the Deoxyribonucleic Acid (DNA) sequence.[1] To understand epigenetics, let's first understand the epigenome and its functions.

Deoxyribonucleic Acid is the hereditary material in living cells. Genes comprise

DNA, and the genome is the total of your DNA.[2,3] Deoxyribonucleic Acid has information to build proteins, which perform various functions. Histones are proteins that facilitate the packaging of DNA into nucleosomes (a part of DNA wrapped around the protein core). Histones are susceptible to modifications that can change the structure or the function of the DNA.[1,3]

The epigenome is a collection of chemical compounds that can tell the genome what to do. These chemical compounds attach to the DNA and can direct actions, such as turning genes on or off – controlling the production of proteins. Epigenetic changes don't change the DNA sequence but alter how the cells can use the DNA's instructions. These changes can be passed on to the next generation of cells while they divide. They can also be passed from one generation to the next. Environmental influences like pollutants and a person's diet can impact the epigenome.[1,3]

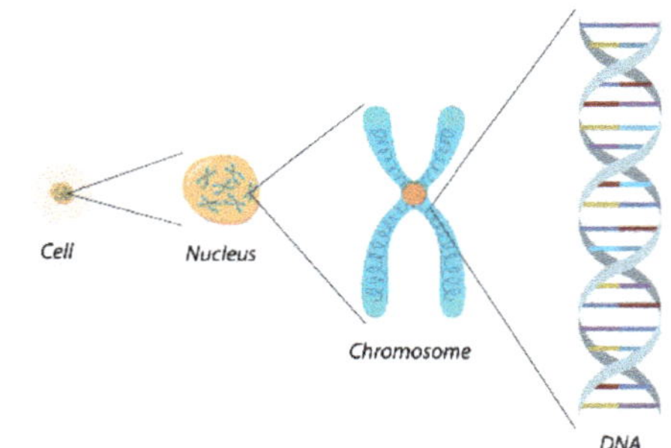

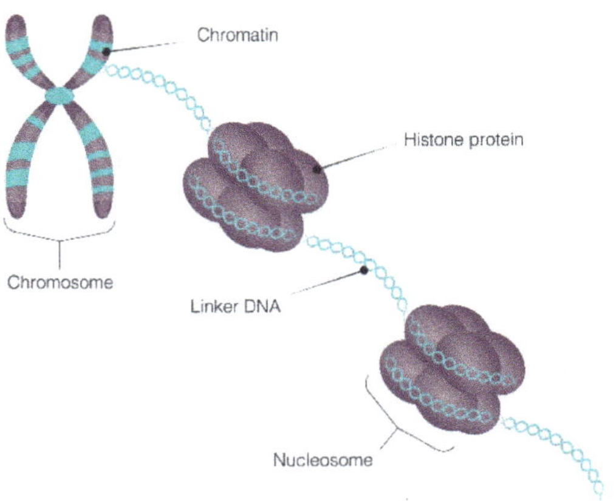

Wondering Why This Is Important?

Your body has trillions of cells specialized for different functions in the brain, bones, and muscles. These cells differ in how and when various sets of genes are turned on or off. One such example is specialized cells in red blood cells that are responsible for making proteins that transfer oxygen from the lungs to the rest of the body. The epigenome can control many of these changes and cause conditions like degenerative disorders, metabolic disorders, and cancer. However, the good news is that these changes can be reversed through dietary and lifestyle modifications.[1]

Developmental Origins of Health and Disease

Developmental origins of health and disease is a hypothesis

suggesting that exposure to certain environmental conditions during important periods of growth and development may significantly affect a person's short- and long-term health.[1,4]

Although many factors contribute to DOHaD, foetal over- or undernutrition is an important one and responsible for metabolic syndrome and mental, reproductive, and mental health disorders.[1,4]

To understand DOHaD, let's take a look at various related concepts.

Developmental Plasticity, Programming, and Mismatch

Intrauterine development is a critical period of plasticity for the majority of organs. Developmental plasticity is the ability of an organism to change its phenotype (visible characteristics like height) in response to environmental changes. If this change is permanent, it is known as "programming." In the majority of cases, programming is beneficial for health. However, "mismatch" occurs when an individual developmentally adapted to one environment is exposed to others. For example, a child brought up in a hot climate will be better adapted to hot climates in later life, as the functioning sweat glands aid in faster cooling down. On the other hand, a child brought up in a cold environment won't be able to cool down easily in a hot climate due to fewer functioning sweat glands.[1]

Thrifty Phenotype Hypothesis

This hypothesis, proposed by Hales and Barker, proposes that severe intrauterine deprivation causes vital organs, such as the brain, to grow at the expense of other organs. These adaptations increase the chance of foetal survival by "brain sparing," resulting in a growth-restricted foetus.[1]

Catch-Up Growth

Compensatory growth, or catch-up growth, is where the child returns to their genetically determined growth for size after a period of arrest or delay. Studies have discovered that this growth is often associated with overcompensation, where the child exceeds normal weight and has excessive fat deposition. This excessive growth is associated with metabolic syndrome, adult obesity, and type 2 diabetes mellitus.[1]

Oxidative Stress

Reactive oxygen species can alter gene expression or cause damage to cell membranes during the critical development phase. This oxidative stress is linked with adverse foetal growth, as well as the risk of metabolic syndrome and type 2 diabetes. Smoking, hypertension, and obesity are known to cause oxidative stress, in addition to being common causes of low birth weight or preterm birth.[1]

Hypothalamic-Pituitary-Adrenal Axis

The altered hypothalamic–pituitary–adrenal axis (HPA) is associated with reduced foetal growth. Exposure to various stressors, such as nutrient restrictions, causes elevated basal or stress-induced glucocorticoid secretion. In a study, steroids were injected into mice throughout gestation; it resulted in reduced birth weight in offspring and hypertension during adulthood.[1]

Neuropeptides

The hypothalamus regulates appetite and body composition by responding to cues from neuropeptides. According to research, maternal nutrition can alter the energy intake of offspring by triggering changes in the hypothalamic circuitry and the action of specific neuropeptides. Various neuropeptides are important in managing appetite, blood pressure, and stress.[1] Figure 1 explains how the concepts of developmental origins of health and disease are interlinked and contribute to the development of various disease conditions.[1]

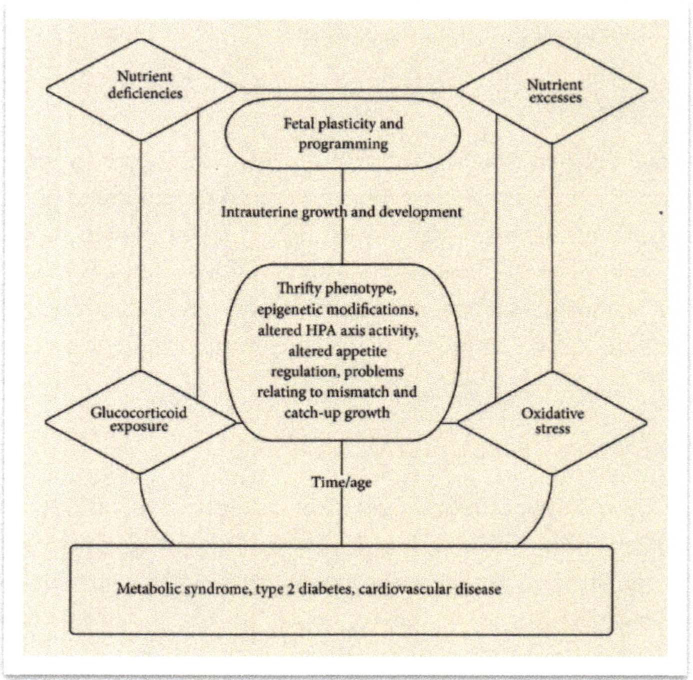

Figure 1: *Relationship between nutrient exposure and concepts and mechanisms underlying DOHaD). Adapted from Brenseke B., Prater M.R., Bahamonde J., et al. Current Thoughts on Maternal Nutrition and Foetal Programming of the Metabolic Syndrome. Journal of pregnancy.*[1]

Right Maternal Nutrition: The Best Start in Life: Now that we have understood how nutrition can influence long-term health, let us understand the role of different nutrients. Nutrients play an important role in maintaining the health of the mother and the child. A list of various macro- and micronutrients and their contributions concerning health are mentioned in the table 1:[5]

Table 1: Role of various nutrients.[5]

Nutrient	Role
Proteins	• Developing food preferences • Fat synthesis • Promote foetal growth
Carbohydrates	• Provide energy
Fats	• Component of cell membranes • Aid in tissue formation
Vitamin A	• Promotes vision, growth, and bone development • Improves immunity
B-complex vitamins	• Energy generation • Development of blood cells
Vitamin C and E	• Antioxidants • Aid in connective tissue formation
Vitamin D	• Maintains calcium homoeostasis and bone integrity

Calcium	• Contraction of muscles • Regulates enzymes and hormones
Iron	• Synthesis of haemoglobin • Transports oxygen to cells
Zinc	• Important components of various enzymes, proteins, and hormones

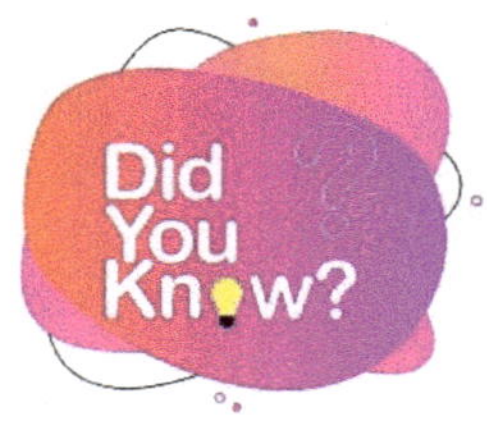

Protect the environment!

Environmental factors also contribute to disease development. Listed below are a few environmental factors linked to disease development:[3,6]

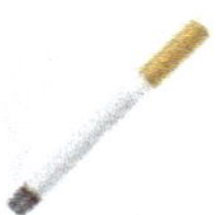

<u>Prenatal smoking:</u> Maternal smoking increases the risk of respiratory cancer, type 2 diabetes mellitus, cardiovascular disorders, and cognitive impairment.[3]

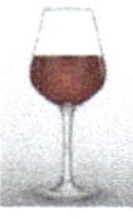

<u>Prenatal alcohol exposure:</u> Alcohol can result in impaired behavioral and neuroendocrine functioning as well as cognitive impairment in the child.[3]

Other environmental factors that influence health are as mentioned in the (figure 2):[6]

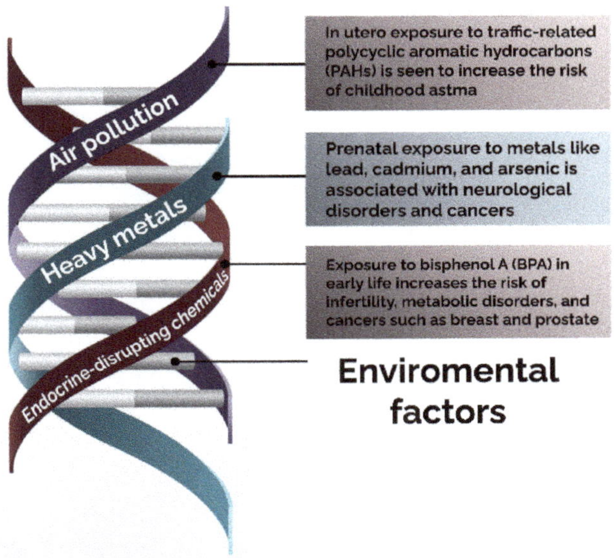

Figure 2: Environmental factors[6]

Don't Wait to Lose Weight!

Your weight, as well as your nutrient intake during pregnancy, determines the genetic composition of your baby. Studies have linked excess maternal weight gain during pregnancy with the risk for various cardiac and metabolic disorders in offspring. The dangers of excessive gestational weight for the mother and the baby are mentioned in figure 3 and 4:[7,8]

Figure 3: Hazards of gestational weight gain on mother.[7,8]

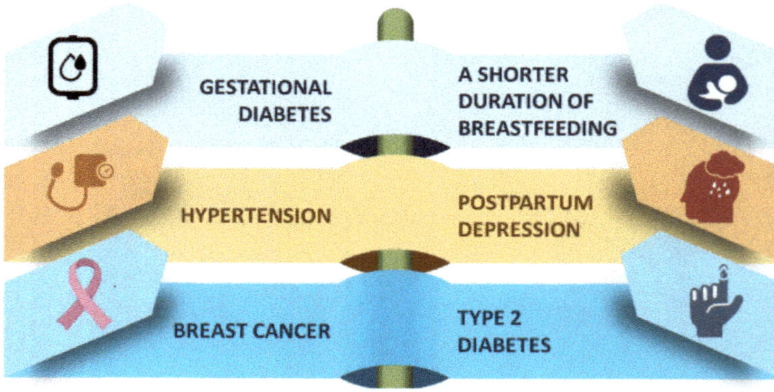

Figure 4: Consequence of gestational weight for the baby.[7,8]

Role of Nutrients in Developmental Abnormalities

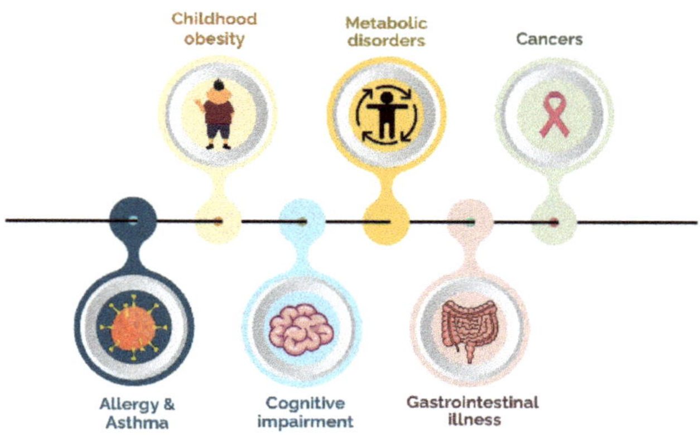

Lastly, restricted intake of macro- and micronutrients in mothers can cause developmental abnormalities in various organs.[3,9] The importance of macronutrients is mentioned in (figure 4)[5]

Figure 5: Importance of macronutrients[5]

Carbohydrate
AS all carbohydrates are converted into sugars, increased exposure to intrauterine carbs can cause metabolic disorders

Protein
Protein restriction can result in small offspring and an increased risk of hypertension in adulthood

Fats
Exposure to high fat diet increases the risk Of metabolic syndrome

Body Composition and Obesity

Developmental programming of the baby can influence body composition by regulating appetite, altering fat deposition and adipocyte metabolism, and increasing the propensity for sedentary behavior. Maternal dietary restriction of calcium, zinc, iron, and magnesium – individually or in combination –causes increased body fat and impacts insulin resistance in the baby.[3,9]

Lungs

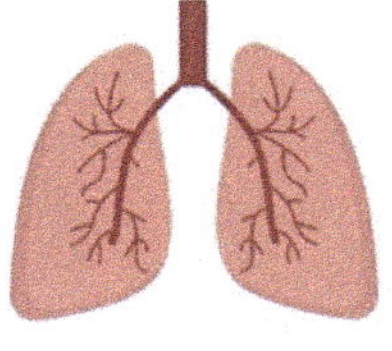

Various respiratory disorders in adulthood originate in the weakened growth and maturation of the lungs *in utero*. The lungs are sensitive to low maternal vitamin A levels. Immature lungs and respiratory failure are common consequences of vitamin A deficiency. Defects in the development of the lungs associated with prenatal vitamin A deficiency are largely reversible with postnatal vitamin A supplements. [3,9]

Pancreas and β-cells

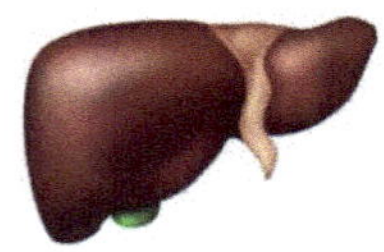

Folate, iron, zinc, and vitamin A deficiency are implicated in developing insulin resistance. Vitamin A is essential for the production of β-cells, and its deficiency causes a reduction in the area of β-cells and glucose intolerance in later life. Moreover, gestational vitamin B_{12}, or folate, status may predict insulin resistance through epigenetic mechanisms. In addition, a zinc-deficient maternal diet can cause alterations in fasting insulin levels and reduced insulin response to an oral glucose challenge. [3,9]

Cardiovascular Function and Hypertension

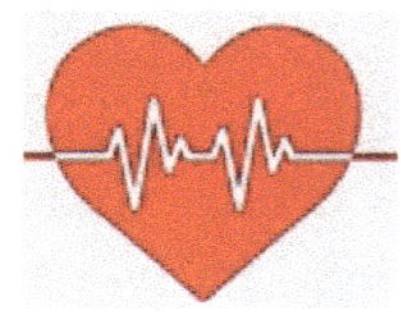

A complex series of events in early pregnancy guide cardiac and blood vessel morphogenesis. Vitamins A and D, zinc, calcium, iron, and folate play an important role in maintaining cardiovascular function. Vitamin A deficiency is associated with congenital malformations. Maternal folate levels can attenuate vasodilation in response to vascular endothelial growth factor and raise systolic blood pressure. Maternal vitamin D deficiency slows the contractile development of the heart. Moreover, deficient or excessive consumption of calcium by the mother is seen to cause high blood pressure in the offspring. Zinc deficiency is associated with altered parasympathetic control of the heart. Lastly, iron deficiency results in hypoxia, which, in turn, increases the heart size and lowers the number of cardiomyocytes (cells of the muscular layer of the heart). It also impairs the development of blood vessels and embryonic hypertension. [3,9]

Kidneys

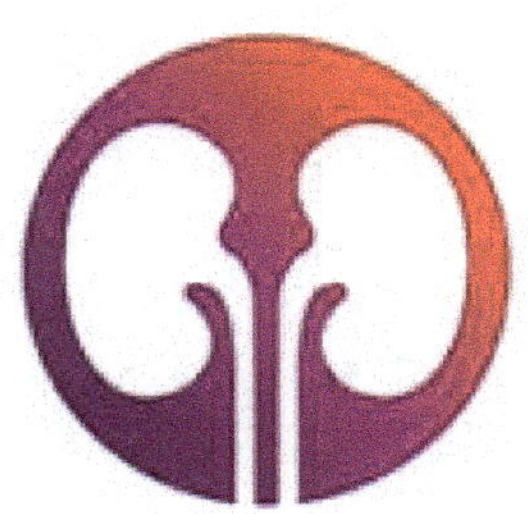

Aberration in the maternal environment can cause irreversible nephron deficits before birth. Mild vitamin A deficiency is linked with a reduction in the number of nephrons. In addition, vitamin D, iron, and zinc deficiency can hamper the development of the kidneys. [3,9]

Neurodevelopment and Cognition

Micronutrient deficiency in mothers also hampers offspring's motor, cognitive, and socioemotional development. Studies have shown that iodine deficiency is associated with cognitive impairment and that supplementation is beneficial. [3,9]

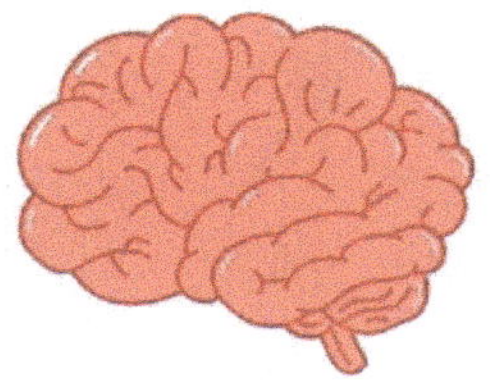

Key Takeaways

- Epigenetics helps in understanding modifiable risk factors for various chronic conditions.
- Developmental origins of health and disease is a new field of study that describes factors contributing to disease conditions.
- Maternal weight and nutritional status play an important role in the development of various organs and in managing the health of a baby
- Restricted maternal dietary intake of various nutrients, like calcium, zinc, iron, and magnesium – individually or in combination – results in increased body fat, as well as having an effect on insulin resistance in the baby, resulting in metabolic syndrome.

It is time to test your knowledge about micronutrients. Match the organs in the 1st column to appropriate nutrients in the second column.

1. The lungs
2. The pancreas
3. The kidneys
4. The cardiovascular system
5. Neurodevelopment and cognition

A. Iodine
B. Vitamins A, D; iron
C. Folate, iron, zinc
D. Vitamin A
E. Calcium, vitamin D, zinc

Answers
1 – D
2 – C
3 – B
4 – E
5 – A

References

60. Brenseke B., Prater M.R., Bahamonde J., *et al.* Current Thoughts on Maternal Nutrition and Foetal Programming of the Metabolic Syndrome. *Journal of pregnancy*. vol. 2013, Article ID 368461, 13 pages, 2013.

61. NIH. What is DNA? Available from: https://ghr.nlm.nih.gov/primer/basics/dna Accessed on: 10 September 2019.

62. NIH. Epigenomics Fact Sheet. Available from: https://www.genome.gov/about-genomics/fact-sheets/Epigenomics-Fact-Sheet Accessed on: 10 September 2019.

63. Mandy M, Nyirenda M. Developmental Origins of Health and Disease: the relevance to developing nations. Int Health. 2018;10(2):66–70.

64. Mousa A, Naqash A, Lim S. Macronutrient and Micronutrient Intake during Pregnancy: An Overview of Recent Evidence. Nutrients. 2019;11(2):443. 2019.

65. Vaiserman A. Epidemiologic evidence for the association between adverse environmental exposures in early life and epigenetic variation: a potential link to disease susceptibility. Clin Epigenetics. 2015;7(1):96.

66. Institute of Medicine. Weight Gain During Pregnancy. Available from https://www.ncbi.nlm.nih.gov/books/NBK32816/ Accessed on: 10 September 2019.

67. Institute of Medicine. Consequences of Gestational Weight Gain for the Mother. Available from: https://www.ncbi.nlm.nih.gov/books/NBK32818/ Accessed on: 10 September 2019.

68. The Journal of Nutrition. Maternal Micronutrient Deficiency, Foetal Development, and the Risk of Chronic Disease. Available from: https://academic.oup.com/jn/article/140/3/437/4600342 Accessed on: 10 September 2019.

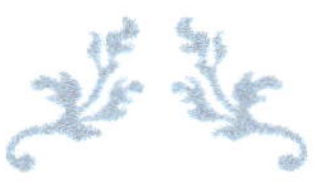

Esha delivered her baby 10 days back. She wants to give her child the best nutrition and, at the same time, wants to shed those extra pounds after delivery. People coming to visit the baby gave her several recommendations about what she should eat and feed her baby. This leaves her confused.

Her doctor assured her that post-pregnancy nutrition is not as difficult as it sounds. If she followed her doctor's instructions well, she would be able to lose weight and consume the right nutrition simultaneously.

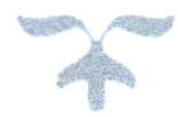

Chapter 12
Post-pregnancy Nutrition

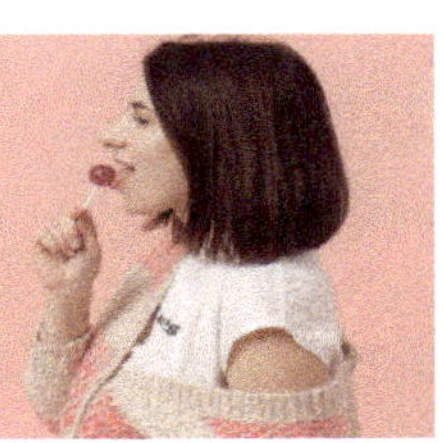

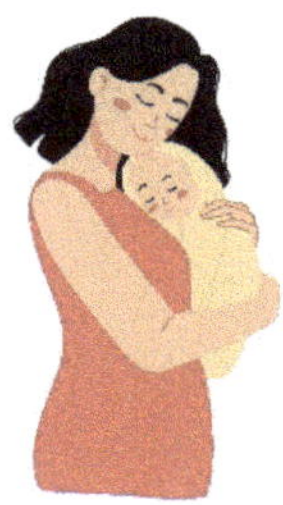

After a successful pregnancy, your hands are full, caring for your newborn baby. A lot is going on post-baby! You're most likely tired, as well as breastfeeding. Thinking about how and what you should eat might be the last thing on your mind. However, getting the most nutritious food is indispensable, as your body works hard to recover from the pregnancy. Getting adequate nutrition might be even more difficult if you have twins or cannot consume adequately. Want to give yourself the right nutrition but don't know how? Don't worry; we have got your back!

Unlock Your Potential With Good Nutrition

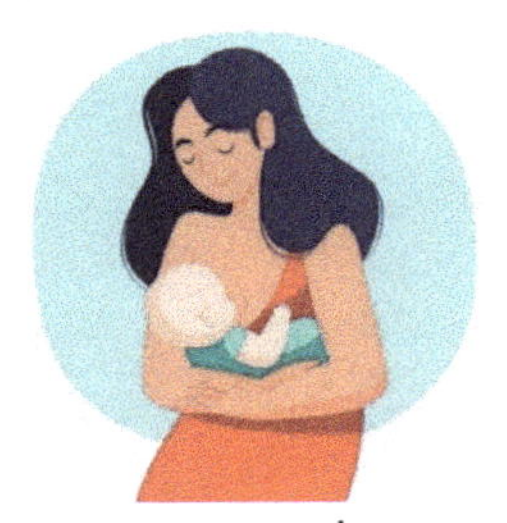

During the nine months of pregnancy, the food you consume nourishes you and your baby. After giving birth, your diet is just as important, as it will help your body recover and provide adequate energy to care for your little one. Moreover, according to research, adequate nutrition in postpartum women can improve subsequent pregnancy outcomes.[1]

Nutritional requirements are different for everyone and depend on whether you are breastfeeding. Majorly several nutrients, like vitamin B_6, folate, and calcium, need to be replenished. Your doctor might advise continuing pre-delivery doses of multivitamins in the following cases:[1]

- Unable to consume an adequate diet
- Carried more than one baby
- Smoking or consuming alcohol or drugs

Let's look at nutrients' role in maintaining health post-pregnancy. Some vital nutrients are mentioned below (table 1):[2–5]

Table 1: Role of various nutrients.[2,5]

Nutrient	Role
Protein	Aids in conserving maternal skeletal muscle
Fats	Essential for the formation of new tissue
Carbohydrates	Balance increased energy requirement for the production of breast milk.
Iron	Aids in the synthesis of haemoglobin and transportation of oxygen to cells
Calcium	Maintains bone density
Vitamin B_9	Aids protein synthesis and cell multiplication
Vitamin A	Promotes vision, bone metabolism, and growth
B-complex vitamins	Aid cellular growth and development of nerve tissue.

Know Your Nutrient Requirements While Breastfeeding

Now that you know the importance of the right nutrition, let's look at nutrition requirements during lactation.

The Institute of Medicine (IOM) recommends the following nutrient intakes for lactating women:[2,3]

Nutrient	Dietary reference intake of an adult woman	Additional requirements during lactation
Energy	Variable	• 500 kcal/day for the first six months • 400 kcal/day for 7–9 months
Protein	41 g	71 g
Vitamin B_1	1.1 mg	1.4 mg
Vitamin B_2	1.1 mg	1.6 mg
Vitamin B_3	14 mg	17 mg
Vitamin B_5	5 mg	7 mg
Vitamin B_6	1.3 mg	2 mg
Vitamin B_9	400 μg DFE	500 μg DFE
Vitamin B_{12}	2.4 μg	2.8 μg
Biotin	30 μg	35 μg
Vitamin A	700 μg RE	1300 μg RE
Vitamin C	75 mg	120 mg

Vitamin D	5 µg	5 µg
Vitamin E	15 mg α-TE	19 mg α-TE
Vitamin K	90 µg	90 µg
Calcium	1000 mg	1000 mg
Iron	18 mg	9 mg

DFE: dietary folate equivalents; α-TE: alpha-tocopherol

A Healthy Diet for a Healthier You

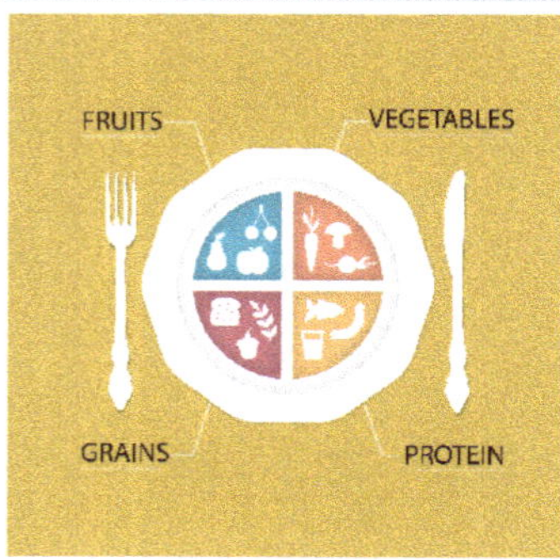

As a new mother, even if this isn't your first pregnancy, you'll need ample energy to care for your baby. Many experts suggest consuming food when hungry. However, new moms may neglect food, as they have too many things to care for.

So, if you want to feel energetic, you should include a balanced diet with all five categories of food:[5]

Fruits: Fruits or 100% fruit juice can be consumed. Fruits can be frozen, dried, fresh, or canned.

Grains: Foods made from wheat, oats, rice, cornmeal, or any other cereals should be included in your diet.

Vegetables: Include a variety of veggies, including red, orange, dark green, and starchy vegetables.

Protein: Try to include lean or low-fat meat and poultry. You can choose beans, seeds, peas, fish, and nuts.

Dairy: Milk and milk products are included in this group. Try to eat low-fat or fat-free products that are rich in calcium.

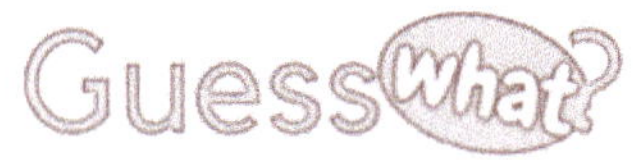

Did you know that caffeine in your breast milk may disrupt your baby's sleep or agitate your baby? The constituents of your milk influence your child's health. Here is a list of dos and don'ts that will help you get the right nutrition, to promote optimal growth in your baby:[5,6]

Dos:

- ✓ Consume more of fluids like water and fruit juice while lactating, to quench your thirst.
- ✓ Divide your food intake into at least five meals per day.
- ✓ If you are a vegetarian, take B_{12} and folic acid supplements, as suggested by your doctor.

Don'ts:

- ✗ Drink alcohol.
- ✗ Consume a diet that provides less than 1800 calories per day.
- ✗ Consume more than 3–4 cups (16–24 ounces) of caffeinated drinks in a day.
- ✗ Eat sea food that has a higher content of mercury. Examples of fish with higher mercury content

Your doctor may recommend a few tweaks to your diet based on the diet you consume daily. If you cannot consume the recommended calories or foods, your doctor may recommend a few supplements. Here's a handy guide to help you meet your nutrient needs: [7]

If you are consuming less than 1800 calories per day	Include nutrient-rich foods that are high in calories. Avoid the use of liquid diet or appetite suppressants.
If you are a complete vegetarian	Consume foods rich in vitamin B_{12} and supplement with 2.6 µg of vitamin B_{12}
If you cannot consume dairy products or calcium-rich foods	Take 600 mg of elemental calcium per day with meals
If you do not consume foods fortified with vitamin D	Consume ten µg of supplemental vitamin D per day

Aim to Be Fit

Usually, a woman gains approximately eight kilos during pregnancy. Many moms experience anxiety about losing pregnancy weight, as we live in a world of celebrity obsession and instant gratification. However, it is best to focus on planning healthy weight loss. You should aim to lose pregnancy weight over six months to a year. Most mothers lose half of their baby weight by six weeks after delivery, and the rest is lost in the next several months. Breastfeeding your baby will also support weight loss. A healthy diet and exercise will help you achieve your weight-loss goals. Provided below are a few tips for weight loss (Figure 1):[8]

Figure 1: Tips for weight loss.[8]

Aim for a pound and a half (650 grams) of weight loss a week. Faster weight loss can cause you to produce less milk.

Do consume the recommended amount of calories. Also, do not skip meals.

Walking is the best postpartum exercise. You can start with a 2- to 4-mile walk around your block with the baby in a stroller.

Factors Affecting Weight Loss After Pregnancy

Weight loss after delivery can be challenging due to various factors, including [9]

- Gestational weight gain
- Barriers to physical activity, like lack of sleep or mood swings
- Sleep deprivation and stress
- Intake of high-calorie food
- Lack of time and support

Postpartum Weight Gain: What's the Consequence?

Wondering what this fuss is all about? Losing weight is not only essential to maintain good health but also to prevent diseases. According to the Institute of Medicine (US), excess weight can hamper lactation and cause postpartum weight retention and postpartum depression.[10]

Long-term effects of retaining excess pregnancy weight include:[10]

- Metabolic disorders: Excess pregnancy weight is associated with various disorders, such as type 2 diabetes mellitus and hypertension.
- Cardiovascular disorders: Postpartum obesity increases the risk of heart disorders, such as coronary heart disease and ischaemic stroke.
- Cancer: Various studies have linked increased postpartum weight with various types of cancer, such as colon and breast cancer.

How Breastfeeding Saves Lives

"Breastfeeding saves lives" and "breast is the best" are commonly used slogans to promote breastfeeding. Breastfeeding is natural, but getting your baby a good latch may take some practice. Try different positions to understand the best position that suits you both. The most important thing is to feed whenever and wherever your baby is hungry. You have the right to breastfeed your baby wherever you want to, and most places are becoming breastfeeding-friendly. However, many moms are embarrassed about breastfeeding in public. If you are one among them, the below-mentioned tips will help you feed your baby in public:[11]

- Wear clothes that provide easy access to your breast.
- You can wear a blanket across your shoulder to cover your breasts while breastfeeding.
- Breastfeed in a sling.
- Practice breastfeeding at home with covering techniques, like using a blanket.

Why breastfeed? Here are a few of the many benefits of breastfeeding for both- mother and the child (Figures 2 and 3).[12]

Figure 2: Benefits of breastfeeding for the child.[12]

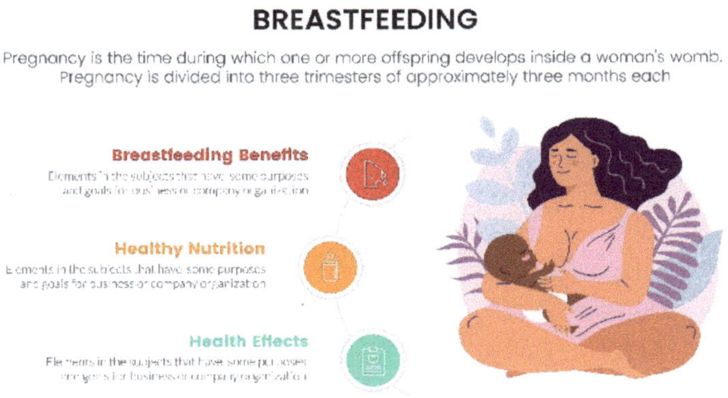

Figure 3: Benefit of breastfeeding for mothers.[12]

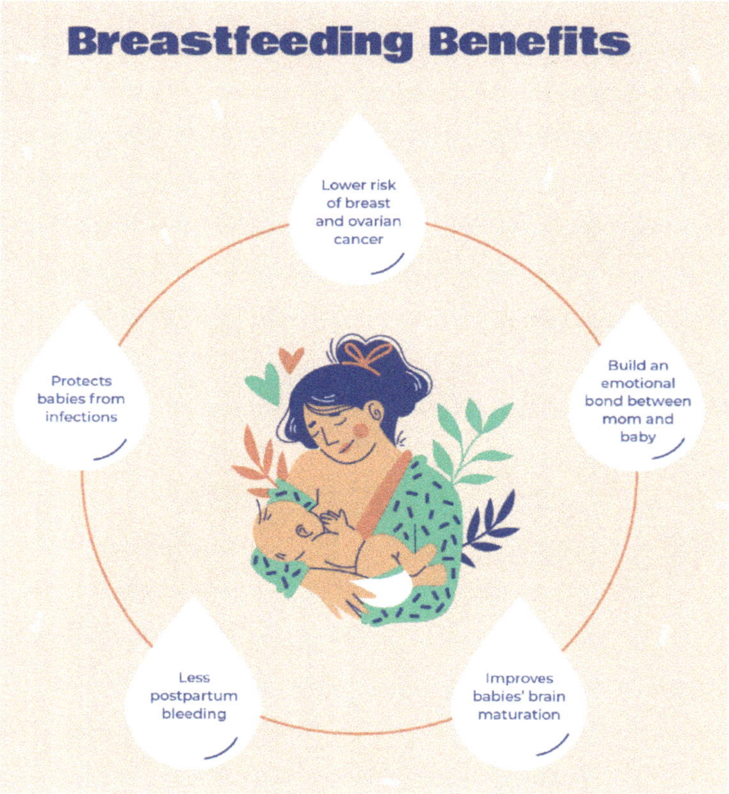

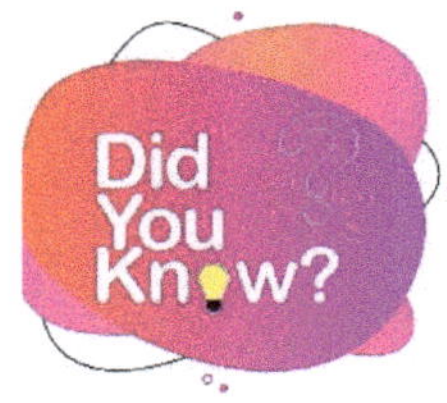

Galactagogues and herbs: Yay or nay

Galactagogues may sound like a complicated word, but they come to the rescue of many moms. So, what exactly are galactagogues?[13]

Galactagogues are substances that aid in initiating, augmentation, or maintaining breast milk supply.

Should I Use Them?

Galactagogues are used to improve low breast milk production in the following cases:

- Neonatal intensive care unit in mothers with a preterm infant
- Infant or maternal hospitalization
- Regular infant-mother separation, like work
- A mother who does not breastfeed but expresses milk using a pump

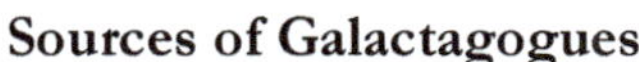

Sources of Galactagogues

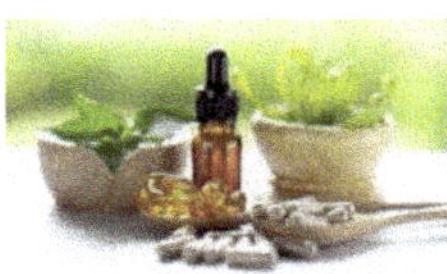

- Drugs: Medications like domperidone and metoclopramide
- Herbs: Fenugreek, milk thistle, dandelion, oats, and seaweed are commonly used herbs.

Side Effects

- Maternal dry mouth, abdominal cramps, and headache are observed with the use of drugs.

- Diarrhea, asthma, allergy, and dizziness are commonly observed with herbs.

It is important to gauge potential benefits and risks before using galactagogues. Also, the mother and infant should be closely monitored for adverse effects.

Key Takeaways

- Nutritional requirements vary between mothers and depend on whether they are breastfeeding.
- Follow your doctor's advice regarding nutrient supplements.
- Do not be hasty while shedding those extra pounds.
- Breastfeeding has various health benefits for the mother as well as the child.

Time to Check How Much You Remember With This Quiz

Fill in the blanks with the most appropriate answers.

1. Usually, about ____ of pregnancy weight is lost in the first six weeks.
   a. Half
   b. One-fourth
   c. One-third

2. Iron needs during lactation are ____ pre-pregnancy levels.
   a. Lower than
   b. Higher than
   c. The same as
   d. Depend on the duration of breastfeeding

3. Recommendations during the postpartum period may include all of the following,

EXCEPT:

a. Small, frequent meals
b. Meals that are easy to prepare
c. Weight loss planning
d. High protein requirement

Answers

1: A

2: C

3: D

References

1. Institute of Medicine (US) Committee on Nutritional Status During Pregnancy and Lactation. Nutrition Services in Perinatal Care. Available from: https://www.ncbi.nlm.nih.gov/books/NBK235913/. Accessed on 2 September 2019.

2. The Journal of Nutrition. Pregnancy and Lactation: Physiological Adjustments, Nutritional Requirements and the Role of Dietary Supplements. Available from: https://academic.oup.com/jn/article/133/6/1997S/4688112#111920813. Accessed on 2 September 2019.

3. Mousa A, Naqash A, Lim S. Macronutrient and Micronutrient Intake during Pregnancy: An Overview of Recent Evidence. *Nutrients*. 2019;11(2):443.

4. Kids health. Pregnant or Breastfeeding? Nutrients You Need. Available from: https://kidshealth.org/en/parents/moms-nutrients.html. Accessed on 2 September 2019.

5. United States Department of Agriculture. Available from: https://wicworks.fns.usda.gov/wicworks//Topics/BreastfeedingFactSheet.pdf. Accessed on 2 September 2019.

6. Eat the right academics of nutrition and dietetics. Tips for Healthy Post-Partum Weight Loss. Available from: https://www.eatright.org/health/weight-loss/tips-for-weight-loss/tips-for-healthy-post-partum-weight-loss. Accessed on: 2 September 2019.

7. Institute of Medicine (US) Committee on Nutritional Status During Pregnancy and Lactation. Nutrition During Lactation. Available from: https://www.ncbi.nlm.nih.gov/books/NBK235579/. Accessed on 2 September 2019.

8. MedlinePlus. Losing weight after pregnancy. Available from: https://medlineplus.gov/ency/patientinstructions/000586.htm Accessed on: 2 September 2019.

9. Goodrich K, Cregger M, Wilcox S, *et al.* A qualitative study of factors affecting pregnancy weight gain in African American women. *Matern Child Health J*. 2013;17(3):432–440.

10. AOGS. Effects on postpartum weight retention after antenatal lifestyle intervention – a secondary analysis of a randomized controlled trial. Available from: https://obgyn.onlinelibrary.wiley.com/doi/pdf/10.1111/aogs.12910. Accessed on: 4 September 2019.

11. Womens health.gov. Breastfeeding in public. Available from: https://www.womenshealth.gov/breastfeeding/breastfeeding-home-work-and-public/breastfeeding-public/#1. Accessed on: 4 September 2019.

12. Dieterich CM, Felice JP, O'Sullivan E, *et al.* Breastfeeding and health outcomes for the mother-infant dyad. *Pediatr Clin North Am.* 2013;60(1):31–48.

13. Academy of Breastfeeding Medicine. ABM Clinical Protocol #9: Use of Galactogues in Initiating or Augmenting Maternal Milk Production, Second Revision 2018. Available at: https://abm.memberclicks.net/assets/DOCUMENTS/PROTOCOLS/9-galactogogues-protocol-english.pdf.

www.ingramcontent.com/pod-product-compliance
Lightning Source LLC
Chambersburg PA
CBHW040140270326
41928CB00022B/3280

* 9 7 8 1 9 5 7 4 5 6 3 7 9 *